T0074723

Geophagia
History, Epidemiology, and Etiology

Geophagia
History, Epidemiology, and Etiology

Anil Gupta

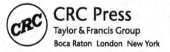

CRC Press
Taylor & Francis Group
Boca Raton London New York

CRC Press is an imprint of the
Taylor & Francis Group, an **informa** business

CRC Press
Taylor & Francis Group
6000 Broken Sound Parkway NW, Suite 300
Boca Raton, FL 33487-2742

© 2020 by Taylor & Francis Group, LLC
CRC Press is an imprint of Taylor & Francis Group, an Informa business

---

Library of Congress Cataloging-in-Publication Data

Names: Gupta, Anil (Child nutrition scientist), author.
Title: Geophagia : history, epidemiology, and etiology / by Dr. Anil Gupta.
Description: First edition. | Boca Raton : CRC Press, [2020] | Includes
bibliographical references and index. | Summary: "The consumption of
soil, clay and chalk by humans is labeled as geophagia. This book takes
a consistent, interdisciplinary approach for reviewing this aberrant behavior,
crafting its etiology, charting its health effects and identifying the universal
traits among the affected population"-- Provided by publisher.
Identifiers: LCCN 2019027537 (print) | ISBN 9780367352868 (hardback :
alk. paper) | ISBN 9780429330391 (ebook)
Subjects: MESH: Pica--history | Pica--epidemiology | Pica--etiology
Classification: LCC RJ506.P53 (print) | LCC RJ506.P53 (ebook) | NLM WM
175 | DDC 618.92/8526--dc23
LC record available at https://lccn.loc.gov/2019027537
LC ebook record available at https://lccn.loc.gov/2019027538

Visit the Taylor & Francis Web site at
http://www.taylorandfrancis.com

and the CRC Press Web site at
http://www.crcpress.com

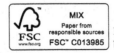

MIX
Paper from
responsible sources
FSC
www.fsc.org   FSC® C013985

Printed in the United Kingdom
by Henry Ling Limited

I dedicate my book to the Almighty,
SHRI SHIRDI SAI BABA

Contents

Foreword

GEOPHAGIA, OR THE DELIBERATE CONSUMPTION OF EARTH, SOIL, OR CLAY, is an ancient practice reported across world cultures. In countries with a high nutritional anemia burden, geophagia represents a major public health challenge. The persistence of geophagia, indicated by its high prevalence despite near-universal condemnation by physicians, indicates the existence of a broad social permissiveness preventing behavior change. Nevertheless, in-depth systematic literature on this subject of considerable importance has hitherto been lacking. This important work by Dr. Anil Gupta fills the gap. The introductory chapter synthesizes various definitions of geophagia, while the second chapter gives a historical overview of the problem. Further chapters explore the prevalence and determinants of geophagia across different continents. Causes of geophagia are evaluated in terms of psychological stress, hunger, cultural, and protection hypotheses. The chapter on the micronutrient deficiency hypothesis provides various evidence substantiating the clinical linkage of geophagia with the nutritional deficiency anemia.

I am sure this book will help readers understand geophagia in greater detail and from a wider perspective, and it will be useful for clinicians, epidemiologists, and researchers...

Dr. Rajesh Kumar
Maulana Azad Medical College
New Delhi, India

Geophagia is a broad term. It is prevalent in developing and underdeveloped countries, targeting mostly pregnant women and children. The author has done a remarkable study in his book, *Geophagia: History, Epidemiology, and Etiology.* He has touched each and every aspect of geophagia.

I congratulate Dr. Anil Gupta for his efforts. This book will help in educating women of childbearing age and thereby reduce maternal and child morbidity due to geophagia.

Dr. Eli Mohapatra
AIIMS, Raipur, India

Geophagia is reported in every region of the world. Although it is a culturally prescribed behavior in some societies, it is also regarded as a psychiatric disorder. Geophagia is a complex eating behavior by humans or animals leading to deliberate consumption of soil. It's a form of "pica," which is the Latin term for magpie, a bird with indiscriminate eating habits. It is seen in different situations and is due to multiple causes.

This monograph is comprehensive and covers different issues related to geophagia, like historical perspectives and the prevalence of geophagia in different regions of the world, and it highlights the ethnic, cultural, and racial bases of geophagia. The monograph illustrates the etiology and different hypotheses in order to understand the exact cause-and-effect relationship of geophagia.

The monograph should serve as a good resource and reference material for undergraduate and postgraduate medical and nursing students, and it will also be a useful guide for students of nutrition science.

Pankaja Raghav
AIIMS, Jodhpur, India

Preface

INGESTION OF FOOD IS A PHYSIOLOGICAL PROCESS among heterotrophic organisms to obtain nutrients for survival. Nevertheless, consumption of soil, clay, and chalk by humans is labeled as geophagia.

Ancient resources and modern references deliver valuable information concerning geophagia and pica in the human race. However, the literature is ambiguous, nonconforming, and inconsistent regarding defining this aberrant behavior, crafting etiology, charting health effects, and identifying the universal traits among the affected population. This book provides an interdisciplinary review of geophagia and is an attempt to put forward a brief conceptual framework to achieve universality in its definition, history, epidemiology, and multiple hypotheses in a single volume.

I hope the book will be helpful in disseminating knowledge about the history, epidemiology, and etiology of geophagia to students, scholars and academicians, and clinicians. I have made sincere and honest efforts to prepare and present a factual book. Submissively, I welcome criticism, comments, or suggestions for the improvement of forthcoming editions of the book.

Dr. Anil Gupta
Dean Research
Professor and Head, Department of Biochemistry
Desh Bhagat University, Mandi Gobindgarh, Punjab, India

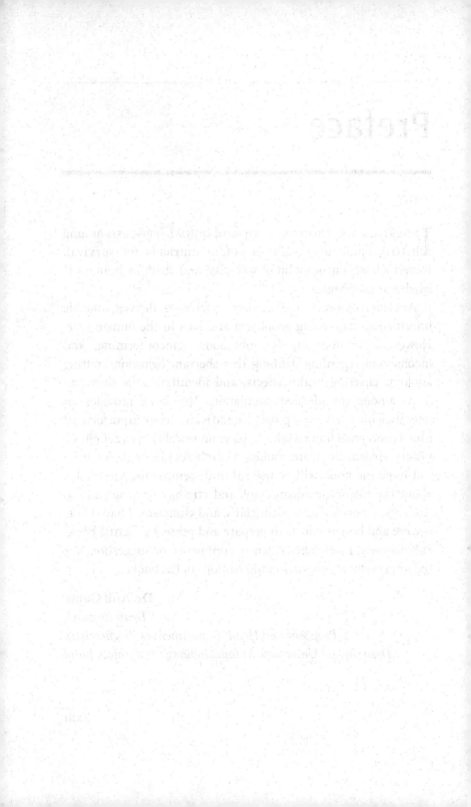

Acknowledgments

THE ALMIGHTY, SHRI SHIRDI SAI BABA, bestows upon me the knowledge and perseverance for preparing the book.

My father, Sh. Ved Parkash Gupta, always inspires me to achieve high goals. I am highly indebted to my parents for inspiring me toward academics since my school days.

I am thankful to my wife, Dr. Deepali Gupta, for her support in data collection, designing the draft, and writing the manuscript.

I am thankful to my daughter, Deeksha Gupta, a student of the MBBS course, for her assistance in compiling the manuscript.

I owe my gratitude to Dr. Renu Upadhyay for focusing my attention toward the Taylor & Francis publication team with my proposal. I am sincerely grateful to Dr. Shivangi Pramanik for initiating and pursuing efforts in the approval of book publication.

I express my thankfulness to Himani Dwivedi and the team of Taylor & Francis Group for their support, cooperation, and gentle attitude toward fulfilling my dream.

Acknowledgments

Author

Dr. Anil Gupta is currently serving as Dean Research, Desh Bhagat University cum Professor and Head, Department of Biochemistry, Desh Bhagat Dental College, at Mandi Gobindgarh, Punjab, India.

He graduated in bio-sciences from Punjab University in 1989. He obtained his bachelor's in dental surgery from University of Poona, 1984. Later on, he did his master's in biochemistry in 2009 and completed his PhD in biochemistry in 2012 from SJJT University, Rajasthan.

Dr. Gupta is presently pursuing post-doctoral research at Srinivas University, related to the nutritional status of children 2–5. He has presented research papers at reputed universities such as Thaper University, Patiala; Birla Institute of Technology and Sciences, Pilani; Punjabi University, Patiala; M.D. University, Rohtak; and Arya P.G. College under Kurukshetra University.

To his credit, more than 30 research papers have been accepted and published in high-impact, peer-reviewed, and indexed journals. During his academic career, he has been accorded merit certificates, merit scholarships, and medals.

Dr. Gupta has more than 11 years' teaching experience, 7 years' post-doctoral experience, and 5 years' PhD supervisor experience. He is gifted with more than 23 years' clinical experience. He is a guide to PhD scholars in universities. He supervises research scholars in distinctive fields like heavy-metal contamination of water, quality analysis of drinking water, and predisposition of blood groups to diabetes mellitus and dyslipidemia. He is serving as adjunct faculty teaching research methodology to research scholars in universities. Additionally, he serves as reviewer and member of the editorial board of national and international journals. His research interests are focused on human physiology, nutrition, and associated pathophysiology. He is an international author of *Nutritional Anemia in Preschool Children* and *Comprehensive Biochemistry for Dentistry: A Textbook for Dental Students.*

CHAPTER 1

Introduction to Geophagia

1.1 INTRODUCTION

Geophagia is an abnormal eating behavior that has been reported among preschool children, pregnant women, mentally challenged individuals, and rarely adults. Astoundingly, the habit has been documented by various authors from ancient periods who substantiate the widespread prevalence of geophagia across different regions of the world. Geophagia has been adjudged a morbid habit in consequence of poverty and starvation, a psychiatric disorder, and an essential practice that is practiced in families and inherited from one generation to another, outside of the culture, religion, and rituals of a society.

Various definitions and conceptual models have been put forward in pursuit of an explanation of the cause-and-effect relationship of geophagia. These conceptual models have academic significance but little interventional role in managing the habit of geophagia. Even though geophagia has universal prevalence among selected regions of developed and developing countries alike, nevertheless, a concrete and collaborative interventional plan against the public health hazard has been completely overlooked. Disparate views have been provided narrating the definition and etiology of geophagia, along with dissimilarity in reporting the types of non-edible items consumed by patients. The ambiguity has resulted in a set of contradictory definitions of geophagia.

1.2 DEFINITIONS OF GEOPHAGIA

- Ziegler (1997) described geophagia as the practice of consuming earth or earthy substances like clay or chalk.

- Danford (1982) described geophagia and pica as the abnormal and intense (pathological) desire for a food substance or non-food substance. In this definition, Danford (1982) included the consumption of both edibles and non-edibles as geophagia, provided the edibles are consumed in an abnormal pattern. The intake of raw rice, excessive ice cubes, and raw potatoes is labeled a pica habit.

- Mosby's Medical Dictionary (2009) defined geophagia as the habit of eating clay or dirt.

- Ekosse and Junbam (2010) defined geophagia as the practice of involuntary ingestion of soil.

- Hawass et al. (1987) and Ghorbani (2008) described geophagia as the intense compulsion to eat clay or dirt or substances from the lithosphere.

- McLoughlin (1987) labeled geophagia a type of pica.

- Johns and Duquette (1991) posited that geophagia involves the incessant desire to ingest clay.

- Reid (2010) defined geophagia as an idiosyncrasy in a small group of individuals or culturally sanctioned behavior related to dirt eating that is widespread across the world within specific societies.

- According to Taber (1985) and Lacey (1989), geophagia is a perverted appetite with an urge for the intake of materials that are termed non-food items that is practiced by a few women in pregnancy through the ingestion of clay, starch, plaster, or ashes. This condition is observable in hysteria, some psychiatric disorders, and helminthiasis.

- According to Stedman (1982) and Lacey (1989), geophagia is an immoral appetite and is the hunger for materials that are not fit for human consumption.

1.3 CRITICAL REVIEW OF GEOPHAGIA

In geophagia, individuals consume soil, clay, or chalk. These are non-food substances; according to the definition of "food" (Encyclopedia Britannica 2017), it is a substance that is essentially made up of organic and inorganic components for use by organisms so as to maintain growth, perform repairs, and derive energy.

Therefore, geophagia is characterized by eating of non-food items.

Eating is a physiological process among heterotrophic organisms to obtain nutrients for survival. Nevertheless, soil, clay, and chalk that are mostly consumed in geophagia are not nutrients. Therefore, eating of non-food items by humans cannot be described as normal eating behavior.

Therefore, geophagia is an abnormal eating behavior.

Some authors have described geophagia as a habit (Johns and Duquette 1991; Glickman et al. 1995; Mosby's Medical Dictionary 2009; Wikipedia 2017). Habit is a regular behavior that is acquired through regular previous practice. Habits are performed subconsciously, as an individual does not require introspection while performing routine behavior. Thus, the etiology of the habit of geophagia lies in the customary practice among certain communities of the world where eating soil or clay becomes an essential cultural practice among pregnant women. This habit passes from one generation to other (Nyaruhucha 2009), while in other tribes, owing to poverty, the habit has been adopted by poverty-stricken people to satiate by consuming soil, clay, or kaolin (Schmidt and Ayer 2009).

Other workers have posited geophagia as a compulsive behavior that is a psychiatric disorder. A compulsive behavior involves an intense urge to perform an activity, unlike a habit, which happens subconsciously (Hawass et al. 1987; Ghorbani 2008; Ekosse and Junbam 2010).

Nonetheless, the American Psychiatric Association considers geophagia a feeding and eating disorder (APA 2013). It is a mental disorder characterized by abnormal eating habits that is detrimental to the health of individuals. Eating disorders are potentially harmful and impair the eating behavior of affected individuals (NIMH 2016).

Geophagia has been reported among women during pregnancy (O'Rourke et al. 1967). It is generally associated with iron-deficiency anemia (Sayers et al. 1974). Geophagia, in the literature, has served to satiate the hunger of people during acute scarcity of foods, as in famine, and could be a substitute for food in poverty (Hawass et al. 1987). Geophagia has been noticed during anorexia nervosa (Woywodt and Kiss 2002).

> Contrary to popular belief, geophagia has been practiced
> in the absence of hunger where factors like environment
> and culture have been strongly implicated in the practice
> of geophagia. (Vermeer and Frate 1979)

Geophagia has been reported as a major health problem in individuals who are suffering from congenital cognitive impairment and psychiatric disorders (D'Eredita et al. 1999). Ingestion of non-food substances by mentally challenged people is associated with a prevalence of high morbidity (Ilhan et al. 1999) and mortality (McLoughlin et al. 1988).

1.4 HABIT OF PICA

The word "pica" is derived from the Latin word "magpie," which is a European bird. The bird is known for its indiscriminate habit of eating various substances, food and non-food (Glickman et al. 1981; Walker et al. 1997).

There is ambiguity over the concrete definition of pica among academicians and clinicians. It has been defined by different authors. Pica is the intentional consumption of non-food substances for a period of not less than 1 month (APA 2013; Young 2009).

Pica has been described as the consumption of either an abnormal amount or type of non-food or food substances by individuals (Kroger and Freed 1951; WHO 1961).

Other authors have described pica as the compulsive intake of non-dietary items for a prolonged period of time (Walker et al. 1997). Pica has been regarded as a hunger for non-dietary substances (Halsted 1968; Lacey 1990).

Consumption of non-food items during pregnancy often involves geophagia or amylophagia (Erick 2012).

Pica is the incessant desire for and intake of substances that cannot be defined as food (Young et al. 2010). It is the consumption of non-edible substances like clay, ice, metal, hair, wall paint, stools, or chalk (Luby 2009). Soil eating, which is a type of pica, has been documented as a therapeutic method to treat chlorosis, which was a disorder prevalent in adolescent girls in the early nineteenth century (Woywodt and Kiss 2002). This pernicious habit has been in practice since ancient times (Laufer 1930). In medical literature, geophagia has been described as a highly prevalent form of pica and an adverse outcome of poor socioeconomic conditions among populations, and generally had been observed after famine and was linked to poverty; nevertheless, the harmful habit has been reported as the intentional eating of soil in the absence of hunger (Young et al. 2010; Njiru et al. 2011).

Pica is common in preschool children and women during pregnancy and lactation. Conflicting evidence has been provided in favor of the practice of pica by the whole community (Bisi-Johnson et al. 2010). Further, pica practice has been found more or less among all human races (Halsted 1968; Reid 2010).

The pica habit has also been reported in psychiatrically and developmentally compromised individuals (Blinder 2008). Studies by some authors (Jawed et al. 1993; Luiselli 1996) have demonstrated that psychiatric disorders are linked with the pica habit.

As suggested by the American Psychiatric Association's *Diagnostic and Statistical Manual of Mental Disorders, Fifth Edition* (APA 2013), certain conditions are deemed necessary for establishing the diagnosis of pica in individuals. According to the APA (2013), the duration of pica, involving continuous eating of non-edible substances for a minimum period of 1 month, and the age of the individual, where such eating behavior is considered unsuitable, are important criteria for determining pica.

Moreover, the American Psychiatric Association's *Diagnostic and Statistical Manual of Mental Disorders, Fourth Edition* (APA 2010) posits that the absence of social and cultural acceptance of the habit of pica is also necessary for its diagnosis, because some cultural groups consider it normal practice, and the last criterion, as suggested by the APA (2010), is that the presence of pica in an individual with any mental disorder assumes a serious concern for the health of the individual that requires immediate attention.

This habit is additionally found in individuals with developmental disabilities (Finucane 2012; CDC 2013; Andrews 1903), which are a wide group of congenital disorders impairing the physical and/ or mental capabilities of individuals. Developmentally disabled individuals have a higher predisposition to pica. These individuals have abnormal behavior that might be injurious to the self and or others in contact with the person (Emerson 1995).

Furthermore, the work of Gonzalez-Turmo (2009) described a new concept about food and non-food substances. According to Gonzalez-Turmo (2009), edibles are liked by people and non-edibles are those substances people dislike, but a substance that is palatable for one might be unpleasant for another person.

Gonzalez-Turmo (2009) asserted in his work that there exists a wide disparity among different cultures in the perception of edibles. It is true that every person has his or her own choice of food items, which is decided by his or her psychology, gustatory perception, access to food groups, and knowledge about foods (Messer 2009). However, the author proclaimed that intake of unusual substances, which definitely have profound negative effects on the physical and mental health of an individual, can never be claimed to be food.

1.5 TYPES OF PICA

A wide variety of non-edible substances are mentioned in the literature. However, the surveyed literature describes the following as the most frequent types of pica habits:

Acuphagia

- Acuphagia is the habit of eating sharp metal objects (Stiegler 2005).

Amylophagia

- Amylophagia is the compulsive consumption of laundry starch. It is commonly observed in pregnancy.

Cautopyreiophagia

- Cautopyreiophagia is the compulsive eating of burnt matchsticks (Thurlow et al. 2013).

Coprophagia

- Coprophagia is the compulsive eating of feces.

Geomelophagia

- Geomelophagia is the compulsive eating of raw potatoes. This disorder is associated with iron deficiency in the body (Langworthy and Deuel 1920; Johnson and Stephens 1982).

Geophagia

- Geophagia is the compulsive eating of soil, clay, or earthen materials (Luby 2009; Gupta 2017).

Hyalophagia

- Hyalophagia is the habit of eating glass particles by humans (Colman 2015).

Lithophagia

- Lithophagia is the compulsive eating of small pebbles and is a subtype of geophagia (Luby 2009; Somalwar and Keyur 2011).

Pagophagia

- Pagophagia is the habit of compulsively consuming ice (Parry-Jones 1993). This type of pica is most frequently practiced by children and adults. Pagophagia is associated with deficiency of iron in the body. This habit is discontinued after iron supplementation (de Los Angeles et al. 2005; Yasir and Glenn 2010).

Plumbophagia

- Plumbophagia is the compulsive eating of peelings of paint containing lead (Mensah et al. 2010).

Trichophagia

- Trichophagia is the compulsive eating of one's own hair. The affected person pulls the hair and eats it (Chamberlain et al. 2007).

Xylophagia

- Xylophagia is the compulsive eating of wood and related substances like paper (Gowda et al. 2014).

Coleman et al. (1981) reported a craving for tomato seeds. Shapiro and Linas (1985) reported a craving for sodium chloride. Marks (1973) reported a craving for lettuce seeds.

1.6 LATEST POSTULATES ON GEOPHAGIA AND PICA

- Parry-Jones and Parry-Jones (1992) and Stillman and Gonzalez (2009) performed a recent study of the behavior and eating patterns of patients. The authors collected historical data on pica patients from the sixteenth to twentieth centuries. It was postulated by the authors (Parry-Jones and Parry-Jones 1992; Stillman and Gonzalez 2009) that pica behavior additionally includes the compulsive consumption of food items in atypical amounts and patterns apart from the compulsive eating of non-food items.

- Parry-Jones and Parry-Jones (1992) and Stillman and Gonzalez (2009) established a new dimension in the definition of pica and geophagia. Lacey (1989), Parry-Jones and Parry-Jones (1992), and Stillman and Gonzalez (2009) cited the 10th version of *International Statistical Classification of Diseases and Related Health Problems* that has been proposed by the World Health Organization and the fourth edition of the *Diagnostic and Statistical Manual of Mental Disorders* that has been recommended by the American Psychiatric Association and stated that pica is the urge to eat non-food substances; however, Lacey (1989), Parry-Jones and Parry-Jones (1992), and Stillman and Gonzalez (2009) additionally postulated that a new dimension like the persistent urge to eat a specific food item has cropped up in the past three decades. Therefore, the authors (Lacey 1989; Parry-Jones and Parry-Jones 1992; Stillman and Gonzalez 2009) concluded that previous definitions that involve incessant eating of non-edibles must be modified through the incorporation of the strong urge to eat an abnormal amount of edible substances.

- According to some (Halsted 1968; Kensit 1979; Shapiro and Linas 1985; Lacey 1989; Ojanen et al. 1990; Anderson et al. 1991; Parry-Jones and Parry-Jones 1992; Fenves et al. 1995; Rose et al. 2000; Obialo et al. 2001; Scott and Cochran 2002;

Stillman and Gonzalez 2009), the definition of pica has been updated and includes both the incessant urge for the intake of food as well non-food substances by humans.

- Ward and Kutner (1999) reported that intake of non-food items is considered pica or geophagia. Lacey (1989) and Ward and Kutner (1999) further commented that the practice of the intake of large amounts of food items like ice is within the boundaries of the habit of pica. Lacey (1989) and Ward and Kutner (1999) commented that the abnormal behavior and urge of an individual to obtain and consume even a food item are within the range of the definition of pica or geophagia.

1.7 CONCLUSION

It is posited that geophagia should be construed after considering the developmental stage, biological needs, cognitive stage, socioeconomic condition, nation's food policy, food security, and, most importantly, cultural facets of a society or nation.

REFERENCES

American Psychiatric Association 2010. *Diagnostic and Statistical Manual of Mental Disorders: DSM-IV*. APA, Washington, DC. Available at: http://www.psychiatryonline.com/DSMPDF/dsm-iv.pdf

American Psychiatric Association 2013. *Diagnostic and Statistical Manual for Mental Disorders: DSM-5*. APA, Arlington.

Anderson JE, Akmal M, Kittur DS 1991. Surgical complications of pica: Report of a case of intestinal obstruction and a review of the literature. *Am Surg* 57:663–667.

Andrews BR 1903. Habit. *Am J Psychol* 14(2):121–149.

Bisi-Johnson MA, Obi CL, Ekosse GE 2010. Microbiological and health related perspectives of geophagia: An overview. *Afr J Biotechnol* 9(19):5784–5791.

Blinder BJ 2008. An update on pica: Prevalence, contributing causes, and treatment. Available at: http://www.psychiatrictimes.com/eating-disorders/update-pica-prevalence-contributing-causes-and-treatment

Centers for Disease Control and Prevention 2013. Developmental disabilities. Accessed 2017. Available at: https://www.cdc.gov/ncbddd/developmentaldisabilities/index.html

Chamberlain SR, Menzies L, Sahakian BJ, Fineberg NA 2007. Lifting the veil on trichotillomania. *Am J Psychiatry* 164(4):568–574.

Coleman DL, Greenberg CS, Ries CA 1981. Iron deficiency anemia and pica for tomato seeds. *N Engl J Med* 304:848.

Colman AM 2015. *A Dictionary of Psychology.* Oxford University Press, Oxford. p. 576.

Danford DE 1982. Pica and nutrition. *Am Rev Nutr* 2:303–322.

D'Eredita G, Polizzi RA, Martellota M, Natale T, Lorusso G, Losacco T 1999. Pica in psychotic patients: An unusual cause of acute abdomen. *G Chir* 20(4):155–158.

Ekosse EG, Junbam ND 2010. Geophagic clay: Their mineralogy, chemistry and possible human health effects. *Afr J Biotechnol* 9(40):6755–6757.

Emerson E 1995. *Challenging Behaviour: Analysis and Intervention with People with Learning Difficulties.* Cambridge University Press, Cambridge.

Encyclopedia Britannica 2017. Food. Available at: https://www.britannica.com/topic/food

Erick M 2012. Nutrition during pregnancy and lactation. In: *Krause's Food and the Nutrition Care Process,* Mahan LK, Escott-Stump S, Raymond JL (editors). WB Saunders Company, Philadelphia, pp. 340–365.

Fenves AZ, Cochran C, Scott C 1995. Clay pica associated with profound hypophosphatemia and hypercalcemia in a chronic hemodialysis patient. *J Ren Nutr* 5(4):204–209.

Finucane B 2012. *Introduction to Special Issue on Developmental Disabilities.* National Society of Genetic Counselors, Inc., pp. 749–775.

Ghorbani H 2008. Geophagia, a soil-environmental related disease. *International Meeting on Soil Fertility, Land Management and Agro Climatology,* Turkey, pp. 957–967.

Glickman LT, Chaudry H, Costantino J, Clack FB, Cypess RH, Winslow L 1981. Pica patterns, toxocariasis, and elevated blood lead in children. *Am J Trop Med Hyg* 30:77–80.

Gonzalez-Turmo I 2009. The concept of food and non-food. Perspectives from Spain. In: *Consuming the Inedible. Neglected Dimensions of Food Choice,* MacClancy J, Henry J, Macbeth H (editors). Berghahn Books, Oxford, pp. 43–52.

Gowda M, Patel BM, Preeti S, Chandrasekar M 2014. An unusual case of xylophagia (paper-eating). *Ind Psychiatr J* 23(1):65–67.

Gupta K 2017. Assessing stunting and predisposing factors among children. *Asian J Pharm Clin Res* 10(10):364–371.

Halsted JA 1968. Geophagia, in man; its nature and nutritional effects. *Am J Clin Nutr* 21(12):1384–1393.

Hawass NED, Alnozha MM, Kolawole T 1987. Adult geophagia— Report of three cases with review of the literature. *Trop Geogr Med* 39:191–195.

Ilhan Y, Cifter C, Dogru O, Akkus MA 1999. Sigmoid colon perforation due to geophagia. *Acta Chir Belg* 99:130–131.

Jawed SH, Krishnan VH, Prasher VP, Corbett JA 1993. Worsening of pica as a symptom of depressive illness in a person with severe mental handicap. *Br J Psychiatry* 162:835–837.

Johns T, Duquette M 1991. Detoxification and mineral supplementation as functions of geophagy. *Am J Clin Nutr* 53:448–456.

Johnson BE, Stephens RL 1982. Geomelophagia. An unusual pica in iron-deficiency anemia. *Am J Med* 73(6):931–932.

Kensit M 1979. Appetite disturbances in dialysis patients. *J Am Assoc Nephrol Nurses Tech* 6(4):194–199.

Kroger WS, Freed SC 1951. *Psychosomatic Gynaecology.* Saunders, Philadelphia.

Lacey EP 1989. Pica: Consideration of a historical and current problem with racial/ethnic/cultural overtones. *Explor Ethn Stud* 12(1). Available at: https://scholarscompass.vcu.edu/cgi/viewcontent.cgi?article=1381&context=ees

Lacey EP 1990. Broadening the perspective of pica: Literature review: *Public Health Rep* 105:29–35.

Langworthy CF, Deuel HJ Jr 1920. *Digestibility of Raw Corn, Potato, and Wheat Starches* (From the Office of Home Economics, States Relations Service, United States Department of Agriculture, Washington).

Laufer B 1930. *Geophagy: Anthropological Series.* Field Museum of Natural History, Chicago, Vol. 18, no. 2, pp. 99–198.

de Los Angeles L, de Tournemire R, Alvin P 2005. Pagophagia: Pica caused by iron deficiency in an adolescent. *Arch Pediatr* 12(2):215–217.

Luby JL (editor) 2009. *Handbook of Preschool Mental Health: Development, Disorders, and Treatment.* Guilford Press, New York, pp. 129.

Luiselli JK 1996. Pica as obsessive-compulsive disorder. *J Behav Ther Exp Psychiatry* 27:195–196.

Marks JW 1973. Lettuce craving and iron deficiency. *Ann Int Med* 9:612.

McLoughlin IJ 1987. The pica habit. *Hosp Med* 37:289–290.

McLoughlin IJ 1988. Pica as a cause of death in three mentally handicapped men. *Br J Psychiatry* 152:842–845.

Mensah FO, Twumasi P, Amenawonyo XK, Larbie C, Jnr AK 2010. Pica practice among pregnant women in the Kumasi metropolis of Ghana. *Int Health* 2(4):282–286.

Mac Clancy J, Jeya Henry C, Macbeth H (editors) 2009. Food definitions and boundaries. Eating constrains and human identities. In: *Consuming the Inedible: Neglected Dimensions of Food Choice.* Berghahn Books, New York.

Mosby's Medical Dictionary 2009. Meaning of Geophagia. Available at: http://medical-dictionary.thefreedictionary.com/geophagia

National Institute of Mental Health 2016. Definition of Eating Disorder. Available at: https://www.nimh.nih.gov/health/topics/eating-disorders/index.shtml

Njiru H, Elchalal U, Paltiel O 2011. Geophagy during pregnancy in Africa: A literature review. *Obstet Gynecol Surv* 66(7):452–459.

Nyaruhucha CN 2009. Food cravings, aversions and pica among pregnant women in Dar es Salaam, Tanzania. *Tanzan J Health Res* 11(1):29–34.

Obialo CI, Crowell AK, Wen XJ, Conner AC, Simmons EL 2001. Clay pica has no hematologic or metabolic correlate in chronic hemodialysis patients. *J Ren Nutr* 11(1):32–36.

Ojanen S, Oksa H, Pasternac A 1990. Pica in renal patients. *Dial Transplant* 19:429–433.

O'Rourke DE, Quinn JG, Nicholson JO, Gibson HH 1967. Geophagia during pregnancy. *Obstet Gynecol* 29:581–584.

Parry-Jones B 1993. Pagophagia, or compulsive ice consumption: A historical perspective. *Psychol Med* 22(3):561–571.

Parry-Jones B, Parry-Jones WL 1992. Pica: Symptom or eating disorder? *Br J Psychiatry* 160:341–354.

Reid RM 2010. Cultural and medical perspective on geophagia. *Med Anthropol* 13:337–351.

Rose EA, Porcerelli JH, Neale AV 2000. Pica: Common but commonly missed. *J Am Board Fam Pract* 13(5):353–358.

Sayers G, Lipschitz DA, Sayers M, Seftel HC, Bothwell TH, Charlton RW 1974. Relationship between pica and iron nutrition in Johannesburg black adults. *S Afr Med J* 68:1655–1660.

Schmidt B, Ayer A 2009. Dirt poor Haitians eat mud cookies to survive. Huffington Post.

Scott C, Cochran S 2002. Pica through the ages. *Renalink* 3(1):7–9.

Shapiro MO, Linas SL 1985. Sodium chloride pica secondary to iron deficiency anemia. *Am J Kidney Dis* 5:67–68.

Somalwar A, Keyur KD 2011. Lithophagia: Pebbles in and pebbles out. *J Assoc Physicians India* 59:170.

Stedman TL (1982). *Illustrated Stedman's Medical Dictionary.* 24th edition, Williams and Wilkins, Baltimore.

Stiegler LN 2005. Understanding pica behavior: A review for clinical and education professionals. *Focus on Autism and Other Developmental Disabilities* 20(1):27–38.

Stillman MA, Gonzalez EA 2009. The incidence of pica in a sample of dialysis patients. *J Psychol Couns* 1(5):066–093.

Taber CW (1985) *Taber's Cyclopedic Medical Dictionary.* F.A. Davis, Philadelphia.

Thurlow JS, Little DJ, Baker TP, Yuan CM 2013. Possible potassium chlorate nephrotoxicity associated with chronic matchstick ingestion. *Clin Kidney J* 6(3):316–318.

Vermeer DE, Frate DA 1979. Geophagia in rural Mississippi: Environmental and cultural contexts and nutritional implications. *Am J Clin Nutr* 32:2129–2135.

Walker ARP, Walker BF, Sookaria FI, Cannan RJ 1997. Pica. *J R Soc Health* 117(5):280–284.

Ward P, Kutner NG 1999. Reported pica behavior in a sample of incident dialysis patients. *J Ren Nutr* 9(1):14–20.

Wikipedia, The Free Encyclopedia 2017. Geophagia. Available at: https://en.wikipedia.org/wiki/Geophagia

World Health Organization 1961. Expert committee on maternal and child health. Public health aspects of low birth-weight. In: *Maternal Nutrition and the Course of Pregnancy.* Food and Nutrition Board 1971. National Academy of Science, Washington, DC.

Woywodt A, Kiss A 2002. Geophagia: The history of earth-eating. *J R Soc Med* 95:143–146.

Yasir K, Glenn T 2010. Pica in iron deficiency: A case series. *J Med Case Reports* 4:86.

Young SL 2009. Evidence for the consumption of the inedible. In: *Consuming the Inedible. Neglected Dimensions of Food Choice,* MacClancy J, Henry J, Macbeth H (editors). Berghahn Books, Oxford, pp. 17–30.

Young SL, Khalfan SS, Farag TH, Kavle JA, Ali SM, Hajji H, Rasmussen KM, Pelto GH, Tielsch JM, Stolzfus RJ 2010. Association of pica with anemia and gastrointestinal distress among pregnant women in Zanzibar, Tanzania. *Am J Trop Med Hyg* 83(1):144–151.

Ziegler J 1997. Geophagia: A vestige of paleonutrition? *Trop Med Int Health* 2(7):609–611.

CHAPTER 2

History of Geophagia

2.1 INTRODUCTION

Geophagia is a universally permeating health hazard of the human population. It has been practiced since prehistoric time periods for which little literary evidence is available. The writings of priests, physicians, philosophers, and travelers in ancient, medieval, and cotemporary periods are rich literary evidence that proves the universal nature of the habit of geophagia.

2.2 PREHISTORIC EVIDENCE

Geophagia among humans is archaic. Its habitude corresponds to the beginning of human civilization. Prehistoric time is a huge period about which archaeologists and anthropologists can make tentative declarations. The foremost evidence of geophagia belongs to the early Pleistocene period. It is the white clay enriched with calcium that has been discovered together with the bones of *Homo habilis* from Kalambo Falls, which is an archaeological site around 30 kilometers northwest of the Mbala district of Zambia, on the border of Zambia and Tanzania (Abrahams 2013; UNESCO 2017; Wikipedia 2017a). *Homo habilis* was the immediate ancestor of *Homo sapiens*, modern man. *Homo habilis* are now nonexistent; however, the habit of geophagia is still prevalent, which is indicative of the adaptive nature of the behavior.

It was Prof. John Desmond Clark who excavated in the lake beds during the period between 1956 and 1959 and revealed a stone-age inhabitation.

> This fact substantiates that our ancestors were consuming clay around 2.8 million years ago in the evolutionary history of humans.

Conclusion:

> Geophagia is universally practiced by pregnant women, preschool children, developmentally challenged individuals in rural populations, urban populations, tribal and nomadic populations except documentation of any cases of geophagia in Japan (Abrahams 2013).

2.3 ANCIENT HISTORICAL EVIDENCE

The earliest ancient historical evidence dates back to around 2500 BC. Medicinal clay was used in ancient Mesopotamia (a historical region that corresponds to Kuwait, Syria, and Iraq) (BBC 2019; Wikipedia 2019a). The clay was sold in the form of tablets.

According to some (Williams and Haydel 2008; Richard 2013; Wikipedia 2019a), the ancient Egyptians in the period between 3000 and 2500 BC were also familiar with the use of clay. During this period, the pharaohs had a strong hold over the Egyptian people. The pharaohs, acting as physicians, used clay due to its anti-infective and anti-inflammatory properties. Richard (2013), and Wikipedia (2019a) reported the use of clay in preparing mummies. Margaret (2008), Richard (2013), and Wikipedia (2019a) also mentioned the use of clay in the Egyptian period by Cleopatra (the Egyptian ruler) for her body massage and detoxification.

Ebbell et al. (1937) and Wikipedia (2019b) mentioned an Egyptian medical treatise that contained knowledge about herbs.

It dates back to around 1550 BC. This treatise mentioned the use of clay for various medicinal properties in Egypt.

The textbook of Hippocrates , divulges perceptive knowledge about the practice of geophagia. Hippocrates was a Greek physician during the period between 460 and 370 BC. He was the first physician who declared that diseases are not due to curses of the gods, and he propounded a causative theory of diseases.

Hippocrates mentioned "ill effects over the head of a newborn baby whose mother consumed pica during pregnancy" (Hippocrates 1839; Danford 1982; Walker et al. 1997).

The medical textbook of Hippocrates was highly regarded among Roman and Greek physicians. Therefore, the practice of geophagia among the population during ancient times was well known in the medical fraternity.

Woywodt and Kiss (2002) mentioned in their article another popular Roman medical textbook called *De Medicina*. Aulus Cornelius Celsus (14–37 AD) compiled the book. He was an encyclopedist (Wikipedia 2017a). The medical textbook portrays a vivid account of diet, drugs, and surgery that were practiced during ancient periods.

According to an English translation of *De Medicina* by Spencer (1971), the book mentions, according to Woywodt and Kiss (2002):

> In the absence of jaundice, bad color of skin of persons is either due to pains in the head or to the tendency of earth eating.

This statement in *De Medicina* mentions color of skin as a manifestation of anemia and, moreover, undeniably postulated a correlation between anemia and geophagia.

A Roman philosopher, Gaius Plinius Secundus, was a prolific writer in the period between 23 and 79 AD (Wikipedia 2017). He wrote an encyclopedia called *Naturalis Historia*.

Pliny described the soil of Lemnos, an island of Greece, as being considered sacred, and it was consumed by the inhabitants (Abrahams 2013).

Woywodt and Kiss (2002) mentioned another memoir of Pliny. According to the authors, he cited the use of "alica," which was a porridge-like cereal containing red clay as an important constituent.

> Pliny commented, "Consumed as a drug with its soothing effect, used a panacea for ulcers in moist body parts like mouth or anus. Also used as enema to arrest diarrhoea, when taken via mouth, it controls menstruation." (Pliny 1972; Woywodt and Kiss 2002)

During the period between 98 and 138AD, the Roman physician Soranus mentioned the use of geophagia among pregnant women. According to Callahan (2000), Soranus described the utility of geophagia to overcome a strong appetite for unusual substances. He mentioned the 40th day after pregnancy, in which women expressed a desire to engage in geophagia. The author asserted that Soranus was thoroughly aware of the ill effects of geophagia materials consumed during pregnancy by women.

Moreover, an alternative narrative was provided by Aetius of Amida in his compilation during the sixth century. He mentioned geophagia in the Byzantine era. Aetius was a physician in the court of Emperor Justinian in Constantinople.

According to Woywodt and Kiss (2002), Aetius wrote:

> Tentatively, in the 2nd month of pregnancy, a disorder arises which has been termed "pica", its name taken from a living bird, "magpie". Pregnant women crave different objects; some ask for spicy objects, while others desire salty preparations, still others ashes, eggshells or earth. (Wegscheider 1901; Coltman 1969)

2.4 MEDIEVAL HISTORICAL EVIDENCE

The Persian thinker Ibn Sina, who lived during the period 980–1037 AD, was also called Avicenna. He was the most famous writer on philosophy and medicine. He collected and compiled a medical treatise called *The Canon of Medicine* (Wikipedia 2017b, Wikipedia 2017c).

The book was highly regarded in the field of medicine. It described the practice of geophagia among children and women. Ibn Sina advocated imprisonment as a method to stop the habit of geophagia among young children, according to Rosselle (1970) and Woywodt and Kiss (2002).

In medieval Europe, some medical texts were written in the southwestern Italian city Salerno attributed to Trotula of Salerno (Wikipedia 2017d). The texts were named the *Book on Conditions of Women*, *Book of Women's Cosmetics*, and *Book of Treatments for Women* (Wikipedia 2017c). In twelfth-century Europe, Salerno was recognized as a center for delivering Arabic medicine to the countries of Europe (Benton 1985).

The texts described geophagia among pregnant women and recommended treatment for the same. Trotula of Salerno mentioned:

> But if she would desire for potter's earth or chalk or coals, then beans cooked with sugar should be given to her.
> (Mason-Hohl 1940; Salerno 2001; Woywodt and Kiss 2002)

2.5 CONTEMPORARY EVIDENCE

During the sixteenth century in Europe, the disease chlorosis manifested among adolescent girls. It was also called the "green disease." The exact nature of the disease was not understood; however, it essentially had anemia as a clinical feature. According to Parry-Jones and Parry-Jones (1992), "It was presumed that geophagia was associated with chlorosis among girls."

Ledelius (1668) speculated about the etiology and pathogenesis of geophagia. He asserted that undigested food in the stomach putrefied there. It became the prime reason for an altered sense of taste and hence manifested as a craving for non-food substances.

Deutch (1977) and Starks and Slabach (2012) posited that geophagia was in practice during the eighteenth century. They mentioned the sultan of Turkey, who consumed clay that was obtained from the island of Lemnos. This clay had a status of healthy food among Europeans.

Vermeer and Frate (1979) made an account of geophagia practiced by slaves in Africa.

Halsted (1968) described the observations of Alexander von Humboldt, a Prussian geographer and naturalist. He narrated a customary practice among the Otomacs during his journeys in the period around 1799–1800. The Otomacs represent an extinct aboriginal group of southern Venezuela (Merriam Webster 2017):

> Otomacs had a habit of eating large amounts of soil and mothers fed clay to their children in order to pacify them.

Another work by John and Thomas (1833) gave exhaustive information about the physique of Otomacs, their activities, and their voracious clay-eating habit. The work described that the Otomacs used to eat fine clay of a yellow color. Clay was collected from river beds and was slightly baked to change its color to reddish owing to the presence of iron oxide. Balls of clay were heaped up in the form of pyramids in huts. Children, women, and adults had a voracious craving for clay eating, as described by the authors in the book *The Mirror of Literature, Amusement and Instructions* in the chapter "Earth Eaters in South America" by Baron von Humboldt.

Hawass et al. (1987) and Hunter (1993) described in their articles the work of missionaries who traveled in Africa in the eighteenth century. They described the ingestion of clay.

Since past history, scarce literature on geophagia has been published. A few available studies have indicated its association with poor socioeconomic background, especially given that the condition became worse in developing countries (Simon 1998).

Travelers and missionaries in Africa also reported the practice of geophagia during the eighteenth to twentieth centuries in countries like Nigeria, Ghana, and Sierra-Leone (Hunter 1993).

2.6 SUMMARY

- The foremost evidence of geophagia belonged to the early Pleistocene period. It was the white clay enriched with calcium that has been discovered together with the bones of *Homo habilis* from Kalambo Falls, which is an archaeological site around 30 kilometers northwest of the Mbala district of Zambia, on the border of Zambia and Tanzania.

- Our ancestors were consuming clay around 2.8 million years ago in the evolutionary history of humans.

- The earliest ancient historical evidence dates back to around 2500 BC. Medicinal clay was used in ancient Mesopotamia. The clay was sold in the form of tablets.

- A textbook of Hippocrates, the oldest written manuscript, divulges perceptive knowledge about the practice of geophagia. Hippocrates was a Greek physician during the period between 460 and 370 BC. He was the first physician who declared that diseases are not due to a curse of the gods and propounded the causative theory of diseases.

- Another popular Roman medical textbook was *De Medicina*. Aulus Cornelius Celsus (14–37 AD) compiled the book. The medical textbook portrays a vivid account of diet, drugs, and surgeries that were practiced during ancient periods.

- A Roman philosopher, Gaius Plinius Secundus, in the period between 23 and 79 AD, was a prolific writer. He wrote an encyclopedia called *Naturalis Historia* and mentioned a use of clay called alica, which was a porridge-like cereal containing red clay as an important constituent.

- During the period between 98 and 138 AD, The Roman physician Soranus mentioned the use of geophagia among pregnant women.

- A narrative was provided by Aetius of Amida in his compilation during the sixth century. He mentioned geophagia in the Byzantine era. Aetius was a physician in the court of Emperor Justinian in Constantinople.

- The Persian thinker Ibn Sina, during the medieval period (980–1037 AD), was also called Avicenna. He was the most famous writer on philosophy and medicine. He collected and compiled a medical treatise. This book was highly regarded in the field of medicine. It described the practice of geophagia among children and women.

- During the sixteenth century in Europe, the disease chlorosis manifested among adolescent girls. It was also called the "green disease." The exact nature of the disease was not understood; however, it essentially had anemia as a clinical feature. According to Parry-Jones and Parry-Jones (1992), "It was presumed that geophagia was associated with chlorosis among girls."

- Halsted (1968) described the observations of Alexander von Humboldt, a Prussian geographer and naturalist. He narrated a customary practice among the Otomacs during his journeys around 1799–1800.

REFERENCES

Abrahams PW 2013. Geophagy and the involuntary ingestion of soil. In: *Essentials of Medical Geology*. Selinus O (editor). Springer.

Benton JF 1985. Trotula, women's problems, and the professionalization of medicine in the middle ages. *Bull Hist Med* 59(1):330–353.

British Broadcasting Corporation. Ancient history in depth: Mesopotamia. *BBC History*. Accessed 2019 Available at: https://www.bbc.co.uk/history/ancient/cultures/mesopotamia_gallery.shtml

Callahan KC 2000. Pica, geophagy, and rock art: Ingestion of rock powder and clay by humans and its implications for the production of some rock art on a global basis. *A paper read at the Philadelphia SAA Conference on April 8, 2000.* Available at: http://www.tc.umn.edu/~call0031/pica.html

Coltman CA. 1969. Geophagia and Iron lack. *JAMA* 207: 513–516.

Danford DE 1982. Pica and nutrition. *Annu Rev Nutr* 2:303–322.

Deutch RM 1977. *The Nuts among Berries.* Bull Publishing, Palo Alto, CA, p. 21.

Ebbell B (trans.) 1937. The Papyrus Ebers: The Greatest Egyptian Medical Document. Available at: https://web.archive.org/web/20050226100008/http://www.macalester.edu/~cuffel/ebers.htm

Halsted JA 1968. Geophagia in man, its nature and nutritional effects. *Am J Clin Nutr* 21:1384–1393.

Hawass NED, Alnozha MM, Kolawole T 1987. Adult geophagia— Report of three cases with review of the literature. *Trop Geogr Med* 39:191–195.

Hippocrates 1839. *Oevres Completes d' Hippocrate.* Hakkert, Amsterdam.

Hunter JM 1993. Macroterme geophagy and pregnancy clays in southern Africa. *J Cult Geogr* 14(1):69–92.

John T, Thomas B 1833. The Mirror of Literature, Amusement and Instructions. Available at: https://books.google.co.in/books?id=5vFZAAAAYAAJ

Ledelius J 1668. *Dissertatio inauguralis de Pica.* Christoph Krebs, Jena, Germany.

Mason-Hohl E 1940. *The Diseases of Women by Trotula of Salerno.* Ward Ritchie Press, Los Angeles, 21.

Merriam Webster 2017. Meaning of Otomac. Available at: https://www.merriam-webster.com/dictionary/Otomac

Parry-Jones B, Parry-Jones WL 1992. Pica: Symptom or eating disorder: A historical assessment. *Br J Psychiatry* 160:341–344.

Pliny 1972. *Natural History,* Vol. 9. Rackham H (transl.) Heinemann, London, 285.

Richard H 2013. *Attacking MRSA with Metals from Antibacterial Clays.* ASU Now (Press release). Arizona State University.

Rosselle HA 1970. Association of laundry starch and clay ingestion with anemia in New York City. *Arch Intern Med* 125:57–61.

Salerno T 2001. *Trotula Major: A Medieval Compedium of Women's Medicine.* University of Pennsylvania Press, Philadelphia.

Simon SL 1998. Soil ingestion by humans: a review of history, data and aetiology with application to risk assessment of radioactively contaminated soil. *Soil Phys* 74:647–672.

Spencer 1971. *De Medicina*. Spencer WG (transl.) Harvard University Press, Cambridge, MA, pp. 116–117.

Starks PTB, Slabach BL 2012. The scoop on eating dirt. *Sci Am* 306(6). Available at: http://ase.tufts.edu/biology/labs/starks/publications/PDF/E10.StarksandSlabach2012.pdf

UNESCO. Kalambo Falls Prehistoric Settlement. Accessed 2017. Available at: http://whc.unesco.org/en/tentativelists/868/

Vermeer DE, Frate DA 1979. Geophagia in rural Mississippi; Environmental and cultural context and nutritional implications. *Am J. Clin Nutr* 32: 2129–2133

Walker ARP, Walker BF, Sookaria F, Cannan RJ 1997. Pica. *J R Soc Health* 117(5):280–284.

Wegscheider M 1901. *Geburtshülfe und Gynäkologie bei Aëtius von Amida*. Julius Springer Verlag, Berlin, pp. 11–12.

Wikipedia, The Free Encyclopedia 2017a. Aulus Cornelius Celsus. Available at: https://en.wikipedia.org/wiki/Aulus_Cornelius_Celsus

Wikipedia, The Free Encyclopedia 2017b. Gaius Plinius Secundus. Available at: https://en.wikipedia.org/wiki/Pliny_the_Elder

Wikipedia, The Free Encyclopedia 2017c. Avicenna. Available at: https://en.wikipedia.org/wiki/Avicenna

Wikipedia, The Free Encyclopedia 2017d. Trotula. Available at: https://en.wikipedia.org/wiki/Trotula

Wikipedia 2019a. Medicinal Clay. Available at: https://en.wikipedia.org/wiki/Medicinal_clay

Wikipedia 2019b. Ebers Papyrus. Available at: https://en.wikipedia.org/wiki/Ebers_Papyrus

Williams L, Haydel S 2008. *"Healing Clays" Hold Promise in Fight against MRSA Superbug Infections and Disease* (Press release). The Biodesign Institute: Arizona State University

Woywodt A, Kiss A 2002. Geophagia: the history of earth eating. *J R Soc Med* 95(3):143–146.

CHAPTER 3

Epidemiology of Geophagia

3.1 INTRODUCTION

The geophagia prevalence rate is hard to predict owing to multiple factors that intervene in the estimation of geophagia. Most of the individuals who practice geophagia have their own rigidity of mind, and they claim geophagia is a normal eating habit, withhold findings, and exhibit reluctance that in turn leads to a false prevalence rate of geophagia.

Fawcett et al. (2016) compiled the result of a total of 70 studies and reported that the prevalence of geophagia and pica was 27.8%. They further commented that pica had the highest prevalence in the African subcontinent when compared with other subcontinents in the world owing to the heterogeneous composition of the sample, framed as a limitation of the study. Fawcett et al. (2016) posited that the prevalence of geophagia and pica could increase concomitant with an increase in anemia and could fall in proportion to rising awareness and education in society.

Marchi and Cohen (1990) and Hartmann et al. (2012) reported the absence of pica and geophagia habits in children older than

2 years of age in the United States. Ivascu et al. (2001) and Hartmann et al. (2012) described that around 33.9% of Detroit children in the hospital practiced pica and came to the hospital for treatment of sickle cell anemia.

Geissler et al. (1998a), Nchito et al. (2004), and Hartmann et al. (2012) reported the prevalence of pica in school children as 77% in the African subcontinent.

Geissler et al. (1998), Young et al. (2010), and Hartmann et al. (2012) reported the prevalence of geophagia in pregnant women as between 5% and 56% in the African subcontinent.

Rainville (1998) and Hartmann et al. (2012) reported a negligible prevalence, around 8%, of pica in pregnant women in the United States.

3.2 GEOGRAPHICAL DISTRIBUTION OF GEOPHAGIA

The prevalence of geophagia (pica) has been mentioned by thinkers, physicians, and travelers across the world. Geophagia is the most frequent type of pica among populations surviving in extreme poverty, humans living in the tropics, and tribal populations (Dickens and Ford 1942).

3.2.1 Global Prevalence of Geophagia

Geophagia is an enigmatic worldwide health problem that debilitates nutritional status, behavior, cognitive processes, and the intellectual capability of the affected individuals.

Generally, geophagia is prevalent among children, pregnant women, and persons with developmental disabilities and psychiatric disorders. Its prevalence is comparatively higher in populations afflicted with poverty, illiteracy, and inaccessibility to medical facilities.

Ngole et al. (2010), in their study, described the universality of the practice of geophagia across continents. It has been reported in countries of the African continent, namely South Africa, Tanzania,

Zimbabwe, Cameroon, Nigeria, Swaziland, and Uganda (Vermeer 1966; Hunter 1973; Abrahams and Parsons 1997). Geophagia has been mentioned in the literature across Asia in China, India, and Thailand (Aufreiter et al. 1997; Gupta 2015) and in the population across the Americas (Hunter 1973).

The oldest evidence for its prevalence has been discovered at Kalambo Falls in Africa (Clark 2001), on the border of Tanzania and Zambia. It is assumed by the author that geophagia was widely practiced by slaves in African countries, and this became the epicenter for the global prevalence of geophagia. The global prevalence of geophagia has been witnessed by various travelers, physicians, and anthropologists during different times in the history of mankind.

During the period between 1876 and 1879, a severe famine occurred in the late Qing dynasty in China. It was the worst period in which crop failure deprived the population of food for survival. The natural calamity proved disastrous for human lives (Wikipedia 2017a). It was British missionary Timothy Richard who drew the focus of the international community toward the famine in China (Wikipedia 2017b).

In the writings of Clinton (2009) and on Wikipedia (2017a), the plight and survival needs of the population have been mentioned.

In 1878, Richard made a journey to Shanxi. An excerpt from his diary said:

That persons shut down houses, trade on wives and their daughters, survive to eat roots, carrion, clay and leaves is the condition that nobody denies ... (Thompson 2009)

Kawai et al. (2009) conducted a study in Tanzania among HIV-affected women. It was observed by the authors that about 29% of the HIV-affected women consumed soil.

According to a report by Barker (2005), a prevalence of pica of approximately 25% was found among preschool children; further, 20% (Barker 2005) of pica consumers in the world were pregnant women, and another 10% of total pica consumers in the world were persons with developmental disabilities. Ngozi (2008) reported that the highest prevalence of geophagia has been observed among African countries.

According to another study by Fawcett et al. (2016), the authors conducted a meta-analysis of the global prevalence of the habit of pica among pregnant women. The authors analyzed total of 70 studies involving pica (Fawcett et al. 2016) and described a worldwide prevalence of about 27.8% of pica among pregnant women.

> It was documented by various authors that geophagia's prevalence was higher in African countries in contrast to countries in the rest of the world. The authors asserted that poverty and culture are the prime factors that are inversely related to the prevalence of pica and geophagia ...

According to a study by Karimi et al. (2002), children and pregnant women in rural areas of the city Shiraz in Iran showed the habit of geophagia. Clay is eaten by the indigenous population of Australia, and medicinal value is attributed to clay eating (Bateson and Lebroy 1978).

Bradford (1915) and Callahan (2003) reported the eating of the deep red dirt of Chimayó in New Mexico, which is known for its Roman Catholic church, as it is believed to be sacred dirt with miraculous healing powers.

3.2.2 Prevalence of Geophagia in Africa

Kaolin is consumed in the African continent, which might be cultural or a need to have a feeling of satiety among the poor. Kaolin, according to a report by BBC News (2016), is commercially available for consumption in the markets of Cameroon, a country of Africa. Its intake is higher among women during pregnancy (BBC News 2016; Wikipedia 2017).

Katz (2017) recounted the plight of poor Haitians and supplemented the description of earlier authors regarding the use of cookies prepared from yellow dirt by Haitian poor people. It was the sole source of food to satisfy hunger pangs. The author commented that poverty is a limitation in the procurement of food sources (Katz 2017).

Another descriptive study was conducted by Golden et al. (2012) in Madagascar. The authors executed a population-based survey composed of a total of 760 participants (Golden et al. 2012), which in turn was constituted of 62.5% children, 5.4% adolescents, and 35% adults. The authors reported a prevalence of geophagia of about 54% (Golden et al. 2012).

In a review study by Njiru et al. (2011), it was found that pregnancy was a physiological condition in which geophagia was highly practiced by women around the world, and its proportion in Uganda women was around 84%, whereas, as asserted by the authors, its prevalence was 50% in Nigeria.

Abrahams (1997) and Njiru et al. (2011) commented on the amount of clay consumption among pregnant women in African countries. Pregnant women used to consume a quantity of soil that was equivalent to 14% of the dose of iron that was needed per day in pregnancy (Abrahams 1997; Njiru et al. 2011).

Schmidt and Ayer (2009) reported a clay-eating habit among Haitians, the natives of Haiti, a small island in the Caribbean Sea. Schmidt and Ayer (2009) mentioned the economic, social, and political turmoil with which the Haitians have been overwhelmed and the extreme poverty and pathetic state of the population that have forced them to eat biscuits prepared from dirt, salt, and butter with minimum calorific value, which enable the population to survive in the absence of food sources.

Njiru et al. (2011) cited the works of Saunders et al. (2009) and Shinondo and Mwikuma (2009) in their description conveying that although the proportion of women who practice pica during pregnancy is dropping, nevertheless, the habit is prevalent in about 65% of women during pregnancy in different cultures across the world. Its incidence in pregnant women during the second trimester of pregnancy is about 47% (Njiru et al. 2011), which is comparatively lower than the former prevalence of geophagia.

Furthermore, Njiru et al. (2011) described the variation in the incidence of geophagia in relation to trimesters of pregnancy. Njiru et al. (2011) cited the works of Geissler et al. (1998), Luoba et al. (2004), and Nyaruhucha (2009) in their discussion that the prevalence of geophagia was nearly 44% in the first trimester, while it was only 5.4% in the third trimester; hence, they concluded its highest occurrence was in the first trimester of pregnancy.

Geophagia has been rampantly practiced by children and pregnant women in the African continent (Brand et al. 2009). It is expected to fulfill the dietary needs of the body in hunger and famine. According to Brand et al. (2009), clay is selected precisely for its texture, color, and quantity. Brand et al. (2009) mentioned reports regarding the association of geophagia with iron depletion resulting in anemia, parasitic infestation, and inflammation of gut mucosa.

Hunter (2009) collected information through field study across five countries of southern Africa and stated that geophagia was practiced voraciously by pregnant women, especially in rural areas. A unique fact regarding the source of clay was revealed by the author (Hunter 2009). It was said that large mounds prepared by termites were preferred as clay for eating in pregnancy. The author asserted that it might have a role as traditional wisdom in alleviating symptoms of nausea and vomiting in pregnancy and supplying minerals to the fetus (Hunter 2009).

The habit of pica and aversion to food are common sequelae of pregnancy, mostly notable during the first trimester. A descriptive study was undertaken by Nyaruhucha (2009) on food cravings, aversions, and frequency of pica during pregnancy. Nyaruhucha (2009) selected 204 women in the conditions of pregnancy and lactation from medical centers in Dar es Salaam city, located in Tanzania. Nyaruhucha (2009) reported that around 83% of the women had feelings of nausea and vomiting and asserted that around 64% of women practiced pica during pregnancy and lactation. Further, it was observed that ice, soil, and ash were highly sought-after pica items by women.

An incidence study was conducted by Shivoga and Moturi (2009). The study involved children under 5 years old selected from around 350 houses in Kenya (Shivoga and Moturi 2009). Data were collected by Shivoga and Moturi (2009) through the interview and observation methods. The authors gathered information related to diarrhea frequency, sanitation, and the habit of geophagia. Shivoga and Moturi (2009) reported a prevalence of 37% of geophagia among children under 5. Additionally, it was asserted by Shivoga and Moturi (2009) that diarrhea had a strong comorbidity with geophagia among children in Kenya owing to poor sanitation and unhealthy hygiene practices.

A randomized, controlled clinical trial was conducted by Nchito et al. (2004) on Zambian school-going children in Lusaka to determine the correlation between iron supplementation and the habit of geophagia. Nchito et al. (2004) reported an incidence of geophagia of around 75%, with a significant gender predilection toward girls. Moreover, the authors reported lower serum ferritin levels and a higher prevalence of helminth infestation among participants who practiced geophagia.

A study was conducted by Luoba et al. (2004) focusing on the initiation of geophagia among women in their reproductive period. Luoba et al. (2004) covered 827 pregnant women from Western Kenya, and the study continued 6 months post-partum. The authors reported a prevalence of geophagia of about 45% in women (Luoba et al. 2004). Moreover, additional information by the authors indicated that geophagia declined to a prevalence of nearly 30% at the end of 6 months post-partum (Luoba et al. 2004).

It is not an exaggeration to say that geophagia is rampant and a public health hazard in the African continent. This proliferative practice is attributed to factors like social customs, ignorance, poverty, inaccessibility of medical facilities, illiteracy, superstition, lack of access to food items, famine, and starvation.

This is variously associated with medicinal treatment and spiritual ceremonial behaviors.

According to Twenefour (1999), geophagia is associated with medicinal properties among people of African countries and has been practiced for a long time.

Geissler et al. (1999) conducted a clinical descriptive study focusing on the habit of geophagia among pregnant women and selected 52 women from a district hospital in Western Kenya. Geissler et al. (1999) reported a high prevalence (73%) of soil eating among pregnant women. Additional interviews by the authors revealed that house walls were the source of soil. Geissler et al. (1999) described the feelings of participants about soil eating by declaring that it was considered an essential practice to preserve fertility and maintain reproductive ability among women. According to the authors (Geissler et al. 1999), it is prevalent in Western Kenya that soil eating is linked with blood disorders, the condition of the body, an illness called "safura," and endo-parasites called "minyolo."

A cross-sectional study was conducted by Geissler et al. (1998) on 156 primary school children in Western Kenya. Geissler et al. (1998) interviewed the participants about their history of soil eating. The authors reported a 73.1% prevalence of geophagia among children. They additionally commented that hemoglobin level, parasitic infection, and the prevalence of malaria were higher among soil-eating children (Geissler et al. 1998).

According to Walker et al. (1997), clay consumption has been widespread among women during pregnancy and lactation in countries of southern African like Zambia, Malawi, South Africa, and Swaziland. Walker et al. (1997) reported 38% and 40% prevalence of geophagia among pregnant women in urban and rural areas, respectively.

Others (Hawass et al. 1987; McLouglin 1987) independently emphasized the role of starvation, poverty, and famine, which are highly prevalent environmental and socioeconomic conditions in different countries of Africa, in the pathophysiology of the habit of geophagia among women and children. According to Hawass et al. (1987) and McLouglin (1987), clay eating serves to give a sense of fullness of the abdomen and satiate the poverty-stricken population, although it is devoid of any nutritional value.

3.2.3 Prevalence of Geophagia in America

In a description by Grigsby (2013), it was stated that few publications are available citing the consumption of kaolin by humans. Grigsby (2013) further suggested that it exists in natural deposits in a large amount around the city of Sandersville. While it is a pica material, kaolin is nevertheless an important compound with high adsorptive potential and is an ingredient in the medicine used for diarrhea (Grigsby 2013). In the article, Grigsby (2013) stated that though its ingestion is considered an aberrant behavior, it is frequent among African American women, and its use in pregnancy has been communicated by family members or friends. An academically relevant fact is that consumption of kaolin has been popular among individuals who undergo routine dialysis, as reported by Grigsby (2013).

In the same article (Grigsby 2013), potentially harmful effects of kaolin were reported, including a predisposition to constipation, decline in hemoglobin concentration, and poor nutritional status among its consumers due to its interference in the absorption of dietary iron in the small intestine.

Lopez et al. (2004) stated the difficulty of the underestimated reporting of geophagia among women during pregnancy. The authors said that its prevalence fluctuated between 8% and 65% during pregnancy, according to published sources of information. Further, it was asserted that its prevalence among Latin Americans ranged between 23% and 44% (Lopez et al. 2004). Additionally, it was conveyed that geophagia is linked to iron deficiency and investigation by health personnel regarding its history during prenatal examination is probably underachieved (Lopez et al. 2004).

According to Wayne (2004), a study of the literature revealed that geophagia was practiced by men and women alike and was common among poor populations in Southern America. This practice had its root in the social belief prevalent among society that eating clay helped men enhance their sexual stamina, while it relived the women during delivery from pains and associated complications (Wayne 2004).

The authors conducted a convenience sampling–based cohort study (Simpson et al. 2000) focusing on low-income pregnant women in Mexico and the United States. Simpson et al. (2000) adopted an interview-cum-questionnaire as a tool for investigation. The authors categorized participants into two groups, an Ensenada group and a southern California group, which were based on the places of selection of participants by the authors. It was reported by Simpson et al. (2000) that 44% of pregnant women in the former group and 31% of women in the latter group were used to the habit of pica during pregnancy. The authors commented on the inadequate awareness among Mexican women regarding the ill effects of geophagia during pregnancy.

Another study was conducted by Grigsby et al. (1999) on the practice of eating kaolin in the central Georgia piedmont area. Kaolin is also called white clay, and the authors executed a purposive study by interviewing 21 participants (Grigsby et al. 1999) who were known to have the habit of eating kaolin. Grigsby et al. (1999) asserted that the behavior of kaolin eating was adopted by the natives as a cultural practice and was largely an endemic practice.

However, pagophagia (the eating of large amounts of ice) was reported by Edwards et al. (1994) among African American women during pregnancy from an urbanized population in Washington, DC. Grigsby et al. (1999) reported a complete absence of clay eating; nonetheless, pagophagia was quoted by the authors as occurring in about 8.1% of pregnant women. Low serum ferritin levels were reported among women with pica, and the authors stated that the behavior was related to periods of stress among women in pregnancy owing to the comparatively smaller social circles of the women who practiced pica.

3.2.4 Prevalence of Geophagia in Asia

A descriptive study was conducted by Gupta (2015) on children between >2 and <5 years, who were selected by a two-stage cluster sample method from schools, anganwadi, and slums situated in and around the city of Fazilka in Punjab in India. The study comprised 440 children. Gupta (2015) reported a prevalence of 20.2% of soil eating among children in the 2 to 3 years age group, while it was 1.6% among children in the >3 to <5 years age group. Pallor and geophagy were significantly associated ($p < 0.0001$) in participants (Gupta 2015).

A descriptive cohort study was conducted by Khoushabi et al. (2014) across five medical care centers situated in the city of Zahedan in Sistan and Baluchestan Province along the eastern border of Iran. The authors collected information from 200 pregnant women through the interview-questionnaire method. The sample was categorized into pica and non-pica groups of women. The authors observed a pica prevalence of around 18% among women in their first trimester. Further, the authors reported that clay was a highly favored non-food item that was consumed by participants.

3.3 AGE PREDILECTION OF GEOPHAGIA

3.3.1 Geophagia in Children

Children in the age group between 1 and 2 years have a natural tendency to place non-food substances in their mouths. Chatoor (2009) reported a 75% prevalence of the habit of placing non-food substances in the mouth among infants and a prevalence of 15% in children in 2–3 years of age. Furthermore, Coltman (1969) considered that the pica habit among children between 1 and 3 years of life is physiological. Coltman (1969) asserted that the pica habit beyond the age of 3 years is found in developmentally retarded children. Coltman (1969) estimated a prevalence of pica between 10% and 33% in hospitalized mentally retarded children.

Coltman (1969) suggested that the habit of pica might be prolonged up to adolescence; however, it is uncommon among healthy adults.

Children in the formative years are predisposed to intake of non-food items. Children between 18 and 24 months pass through an oral stage and have a natural inclination to place objects in the mouth and explore through their tactile sense (Ellis and Schnoes 2006; Broomfield 2007).

According to Saathoff et al. (2002), as the age of children increases, the tendency to eat non-edibles automatically declines. According to Geissler (2000) and Ellis and Schnoes (2006), adolescents and adults are generally disinclined to the habit of soil eating.

3.3.2 Geophagia in Adults

According to Danford et al. (1982) conducted a study among mentally challenged adults in hospitals. They reported a prevalence of the habit of pica of 25.8% among mentally challenged adults. Danford et al. (1982) posited that low intelligence quotient was related to the habit of non-food pica in adults. Additionally, Danford et al. (1982) reported the occurrence of intestinal parasites and intestinal obstruction among adults who had the habit of non-food pica.

McAlpine and Singh (1986) stated that the occurrence of pica beyond the age of 18 months is considered abnormal eating behavior. McAlpine and Singh (1986) conducted a study on hospitalized mentally retarded adults and reported a prevalence of 9.2% of the habit of pica among them. The authors asserted that the frequency of pica was associated with the level of mental retardation and age of the patients. McAlpine and Singh (1986) found consumption of dirt, clothes, paper, toys, and grass as pica.

Ashworth et al. (2009) reported the correlation of the psychosocial life of adults with intellectual disabilities and the habit of pica. They reported a prevalence of 21.8% of the habit of pica in intellectually disabled adults in hospitals. Ashworth et al. (2009) posited that lack of interest in recreational programs, poor family life, and poor social links were strongly associated with the habit of pica among intellectually disabled adults.

3.4 PREVALENCE OF GEOPHAGIA IN PREGNANCY

Fawcett et al. (2016) presented data about the prevalence of pica (geophagia) based on interviews with women during and after pregnancy. Fawcett et al. (2016) reported the highest prevalence (44.8%) of pica among women during and after pregnancy in Africa. Additionally, prevalences of pica of 23% and 17.5% were reported in North and South America and Eurasia, respectively, during pregnancy and post-partum by Fawcett et al. (2016).

The ingestion of earth-like substances like clay and soil by women is intimately linked to pregnancy, particularly in India and African countries. This habit of soil eating has been considered to overcome the symptoms of nausea and vomiting, which are prominent during the first trimester of pregnancy among women (Knishinsky 1998; Hunter 2003; Luoba et al. 2004; Grigsby 2004).

According to Woywodt and Kiss (2002), pregnant women in urban areas in South Africa often viewed soil eating favorably for the development of a baby with a fair complexion. Consequently, this habit of soil eating is passed down from the mothers to their children owing to its cultural, social, and familial background (Vermeer and Frate 1979).

Geissler et al. (1999) conducted a clinical study in a hospital in the Kilifi district in Kenya. Geissler et al. (1999) had observed a high prevalence of geophagia among pregnant women. They selected 52 pregnant women from the same hospital in Kenya and interviewed them about the habit of soil eating and its related ill effects on their health. Geissler et al. (1999) found that about two-thirds of the selected women consumed soil regularly. Ingested soil was taken from the walls of their houses. Geissler et al. (1999) reported a strong correlation between soil eating and the occurrence of iron deficiency and anemia among pregnant women. It was posited by Geissler et al. (1999) that soil eating in pregnancy is linked to reproductive power. The habit of soil eating was linked to their traditional knowledge about blood, pregnancy, and fertility.

Roselle (1970) and Crosby (1976) reported the prevalence of soil eating among pregnant women in the Southern states of the United States. Roselle (1970) and Crosby (1976) reported the intake of corn starch, clay, and baking soda, and it was posited by the authors that non-food substances might be helpful in the prophylaxis of nausea and vomiting in pregnancy, and were considered necessary for giving birth to healthy babies.

Ngozi (2008) reported ingestion of pebbles or rock (lithophagia) in Kenya. It was practiced by pregnant women and non-pregnant women, as reported by the author (Ngozi 2008). Pregnant women procured stones that were soft enough to be masticated with the teeth. These stones were termed "odowa." Ngozi (2008) indicated that it is customary in Kenya in local tribes to practice odowa and that it helps women maintain vigor and health during pregnancy.

According to a report by Mawathe (2008), pregnant women have a tendency to eat coal, soap, and gherkins. Mawathe (2008) reported pregnant women with an irresistible desire to eat soft stone, which is termed odowa in Kenya. These stones were commercially available in the Gikomba market in Nairobi, as told by the author (Mawathe 2008). The author described the stone sellers who were in contact with pregnant women for the sale of odowa. Additionally, the same report by Mawathe (2008) mentioned the narrative of a nutritionist named Ndong Alice, who described odowa as tasteless. She discussed in the report (Mawathe 2008) the ill effects of the habit of eating odowa. She stated that incessant eating of stone could injure the kidneys and liver without concomitant intake of a sufficient amount of water.

According to a report published in The Hindu (2015), a reference was given to women in the second trimester of pregnancy in Hyderabad, a city in India, who indulged in eating purified soft limestone, which was commercially sold in grocery shops in the city. This practice, as mentioned in the report, was a custom among pregnant women wishing to deliver a fair-skinned baby.

Another type of lithophagia is in the form of soft yellow stones called "khadi" that were sold in the market by traders across cities like Bidar in Karnataka, according to a report (The Hindu 2015). It was further mentioned in the report (The Hindu 2015) that pregnant women belonging to such diverse religious communities as Jain, Marwari, Telugu, and Muslim were in the habit of eating khadi stones.

3.5 ETHNIC, CULTURAL, AND RACIAL BASIS OF GEOPHAGIA

Although no specific data exist regarding the racial predilection of pica, the practice is reported to be more common among certain cultural and geographic populations. For example, geophagia is accepted culturally among some families of African lineage and is reported to be problematic in 70% of provinces in Turkey. Ethnic differences and societal norms concerning geography, sociocultural factors, and developmental considerations are all significant in determining pica. Demographic information reveals that pica has been associated with diets that are low in iron, zinc, and calcium compared with a balanced, controlled diet.

> Incessant urge for non-food substances is not constrained by any race, religion, tribe, socioeconomic status or gender. It is prevalent among children, pregnant women, developmentally disabled individuals and adults. (Erick 2012: 363)

> Moreover, potential predisposing factors for geophagia include mental retardation, neurological lesions of the brain and psychiatric disorders. (Ellis and Pataki 2012)

> The author hypothesizes that actual data on the prevalence of geophagia are unavailable. Patients are reluctant to reveal the habit of clay eating. Thus, the detrimental habit goes unnoticed. The habit is accorded a social stigma, and this dissuades patients from publicly admitting to the aberrant eating habit.

3.6 SUMMARY

- The geophagia prevalence rate is hard to predict owing to multiple factors that intervene in the estimation of geophagia.

- Fawcett et al. (2016) compiled a result of a total of 70 studies and reported that the prevalence of geophagia and pica was 27.8%.

- Fawcett et al. (2016) posited that the prevalence of geophagia and pica could increase concomitant with an increase in anemia and could fall in proportion to rising awareness and education in society.

- Geissler et al. (1998b,c), Nchito et al. (2004), and Hartmann et al. (2012) reported the prevalence of pica in school children as 77% in the African subcontinent.

- Marchi and Cohen (1990) and Hartmann et al. (2012) reported the absence of pica and geophagia habits in children older than 2 years of age in the United States. Ivascu et al. (2001) and Hartmann et al. (2012) stated that around 33.9% of children in a Detroit hospital practiced pica; they came to the hospital for treatment of sickle cell anemia.

- Geissler et al. (1998), Young et al. (2010), and Hartmann et al. (2012) reported a prevalence of geophagia in pregnant women between 5% and 56% in the African subcontinent.

- Hartmann et al. (2012) and Rainville (1998) reported a negligible prevalence, around 8%, of pica in pregnant women in the United States.

- The prevalence of geophagia (pica) has been mentioned by thinkers, physicians, and travelers across the world. Geophagia is the most frequent type of pica among populations surviving in extreme poverty, humans living in the tropics, and tribal populations (Dickens and Ford 1942).

- Geophagia is an enigmatic worldwide health problem that debilitates the nutritional status, behavior, cognitive processes, and intellectual capability of the affected individuals.

- Ngole et al. (2010), in their study, described the universality of the practice of geophagia across continents. It has been reported in countries of the African continent, namely South Africa, Tanzania, Zimbabwe, Cameroon, Nigeria, Swaziland, and Uganda (Vermeer 1966; Hunter 1973; Abrahams and Parsons 1997).

- In the writings of Clinton (2009) and in Wikipedia (2017), the plight and survival needs of populations have been mentioned.

- In 1878, Richard made a journey to Shanxi. An excerpt from his diary said, "That persons shut down houses, trade on wives and their daughters, survive to eat roots, carrion, clay and leaves is the condition that nobody denies ..." (Thompson 2009).

- Kaolin is consumed in Africa, which might be cultural or a need to have a feeling of satiety among the poor. Kaolin, according to a report by BBC News (2016), is commercially available for consumption in the markets of Cameroon. Its intake is higher among women during pregnancy (BBC News 2016; Wikipedia 2017).

- Abrahams (1997) and Njiru et al. (2011) commented on the amount of clay consumption among pregnant women in African countries. Pregnant women used to consume a quantity of soil that was equivalent to 14% of the dose of iron that was needed per day in pregnancy (Abrahams 1997; Njiru et al. 2011).

- Furthermore, Njiru et al. (2011) described the variation in the incidence of geophagia in relation to trimesters in pregnancy. Njiru et al. (2011) cited the works of Geissler et al. (1998),

Luoba et al. (2004), and Nyaruhucha (2009) and their discussion that the prevalence of geophagia was nearly 44% in the first trimester, while it was only 5.4% in the third trimester, and hence concluded its highest occurrence was in the former trimester of pregnancy.

- Data were collected by Shivoga and Moturi (2009) through the interview and observation methods. The authors gathered information related to diarrhea frequency, sanitation, and the habit of geophagia. They reported a prevalence of 37% of geophagia among in children under 5.

- According to Geissler et al. (1999), it is prevalent in western Kenya that soil eating is linked with blood disorders, the condition of the body, an illness called "safura," and endoparasites called "minyolo."

- According to Walker et al. (1997), clay consumption has been widespread among women during pregnancy and lactation in countries of southern African like Zambia, Malawi, South Africa, and Swaziland. Walker et al. (1997) reported a 38% and 40% prevalence of geophagia among pregnant women in urban and rural areas, respectively.

- A descriptive study was conducted by Gupta (2015) on children between >2 and <5 years of age, who were selected by a two-stage cluster sample method from schools, anganwadi, and slums situated in and around the city of Fazilka in Punjab in India. The study comprised 440 children. Gupta (2015) reported a prevalence of 20.2% of soil eating among children 2 to 3 years of age, while it was 1.6% among children in the >3 to <5 year age group. Pallor and geophagy were significantly associated ($p < 0.0001$) in participants (Gupta 2015).

- Children in the age group between 1 and 2 years have a natural tendency to place non-food substances in their mouths. Chatoor (2009) reported a 75% prevalence of the habit of placing non-food substances in the mouth among infants and a prevalence of 15% in children 2 to 3 years of age.

- McAlpine and Singh (1986) stated that the occurrence of pica beyond the age of 18 months is considered abnormal eating behavior. McAlpine and Singh (1986) conducted a study on hospitalized mentally retarded adults and reported a prevalence of 9.2% of the habit of pica among them.

REFERENCES

Abrahams PW 1997. Geophagy (soil consumption) and iron supplementation in Uganda. *Trop Med Int Health* 2:617–623.

Abrahams PW, Parsons JA 1997. Geophagy in the tropics: An appraisal of three geophagical materials. *Environ Geochem Health* 19(1):325–334.

Ashworth M, Hirdes JP, Martin L 2009. The social and recreational characteristics of adults with intellectual disability and pica living in institutions. *Res Dev Disabil* 30(3):512–20.

Aufreiter S, Hancock RGV, Mahaney WC, Stambolic RA, Sanmugadas K 1997. Geochemistry and mineralogy of soils eaten by humans. *Int J Food Sci Nutr* 48(5):293–305.

Barker D 2005. Tooth wear as a result of pica. *Br Dent J* 199:271–273.

Bateson, EM, Lebroy T 1978. Clay eating by aboriginals of the Northern Territory. *Med J Aust* 25(1):1–3.

Bradford PL 1915. *Spanish Mission Churches of New Mexico.* The Torch Press, pp. 316–322.

Brand CE, De Jager L, Ekosse G 2009. Possible health effects associated with human geophagic practice: An overview. *Med Technol S Afr* 23:11–13.

British Broadcasting Corporation News 2016. The People Who Cannot Stop Eating Dirt. Available at: www.bbc.com/future/story/20160615-the-people-who-cant-stop-eating-dirt

Broomfield J 2007. Pica. *Diseases and Conditions Encyclopedia: Discovery Health.* (Accessed 2019). http://health.discovery.com/encyclopedias/illnesses.html?article=1699

Callahan GN 2003. Eating dirt. *Emerg Infect Dis* 9(8):1016–1021.

Chatoor I 2009. Chapter 44: Feeding and eating disorders of infancy and early childhood. In Sadock, BJ; Sadock, VA; Ruiz, P (eds.). *Kaplan and Sadock's Comprehensive Textbook of Psychiatry* (9th ed.). Lippincott, Williams & Wilkins. p. 3607.

Clark JD 2001. Geophagy and Kalambo Falls clays. In: *Kalambo Falls Prehistoric Site, The Earlier Cultures: Middle and Earlier Stone Age*, Vol. 3. Clark JD (editor). Cambridge University Press, Cambridge.

Clinton TL 2009. *William Scott Ament and the Boxer Rebellion*. McFarland, Jefferson, NC, p. 21.

Coltman CA Jr 1969. Pagophagia and iron lack. *JAMA* 207:513–516.

Crosby WH 1976. When friends and patients ask about pica. *JAMA*, 235:2765.

Danford D, Smith JC, Huber A 1982. Pica and mineral status in the mentally retarded. *Am J Clin Nutr* 35:958–967.

Dickens D, Ford RM 1942. Geophagy (dirt eating) among Mississippi Negro school children. *Am Sociol Rev* 7:59.

Edwards CH, Johnson AA, Knight EM, Oyemade UJ, Cole OE 1994. Pica in an urban environment. *J Nutr* 124(Suppl 6):954S–962S.

Ellis CR, Pataki C 2012, April, 30. Pica. *Medscape Reference*. Retrieved from March 22, 2013 from http://emedicine.medscape.com/article/914765-overview#aw2aab6b5

Ellis CR, Schnoes CJ 2006. Eating disorder: Pica. *eMedicine*. (Accessed 2019). http://www.emedicine.medscape.com/article/914765-overview

Fawcett EJ, Fawcett JM, Mazmanian D 2016. A meta-analysis of the worldwide prevalence of pica during pregnancy and the postpartum period. *Int J Gynaecol Obstet* 133(3):277–283.

Geissler PW 2000. The significance of earth-eating: Social and cultural aspects of geophagy among Luo children. *Afr: J Int Afr I* 70(4): 653–682.

Geissler PW, Mwaniki D, Thiong F, Friis H 1998a. Geophagy as a risk factor for geohelminth infections: A longitudinal study of Kenyan primary schoolchildren. *Trans R Soc Trop Med Hyg* 92(1):7–11.

Geissler PW, Mwaniki DL, Thiong'o F, Michaelsen, KF, Friis H 1998b. Geophagy, iron status and anaemia among primary school children in Western Kenya. *Trop Med Int Health* 3(7):529–534.

Geissler PW, Shulman CE, Prince RJ, Mutemi W, Mnazi C, Friis H, Lowe B 1998c. Geophagy, iron status and anaemia among pregnant women on the coast of Kenya. *Trans R Soc Trop Med Hyg* 92(5):549–553.

Geissler PW, Prince RJ, Levene M, Poda C, Beckerleg SE, Mutemi W, Shulman CE 1999. Perceptions of soil-eating and anaemia among pregnant women on the Kenyan coast. *Soc Sci Med* 48(8):1069–1079.

Golden CD, Rasolofoniaina BJR, Benjamin R, Young SL 2012. Pica and amylophagy are common among Malagasy men, women and children. *PLOS ONE* 7(10):e47129. https://doi.org/10.1371/journal.pone.0047129

Grigsby RK 2004. *Clay Eating*. Georgia Health Science University. Available at: http://www.georgiaencyclopedia.org/articles/science-medicine/clay-eating

Grigsby RK 2013. Clay Eating. New Georgia Encyclopedia. (Accessed 2019).

Grigsby RK, Thyer BA, Waller RJ, Johnson GA Jr 1999. Chalk eating in middle Georgia: A culture-bound syndrome of pica. *South Med J* 92(2):190–192.

Gupta A 2015. Detrimental consequences of the habit of geophagy in children under the age of five years. *Rev Res* 4(4):1–9.

Hartmann AS, Becker AE, Hamptom C, Bryant-Waugh R 2012. Pica and rumination disorder in DSM-5. *Psychiatr Ann* 42(11):426–430.

Hawass NED, Alnozha MM, Kolawole T 1987. Adult geophagia—report of three cases with review of the literature. *Trop Geogr Med* 39: 191–5

Hunter JM 1973. Geophagy in Africa and the United States: Culture-nutrition hypothesis. *Geogr Rev* 63:170–195.

Hunter BT 2003. The Widespread Practice of Consuming Soil. Consumer's Research Magazine. (Accessed 2019). http://www.highbeam.com/doc/1G1-112542811.html

Hunter JM 2009. Macroterme geophagy and pregnancy clays in southern Africa. *J Cult Geogr* 14(1):69–92.

Ivascu NS, Sarnaik S, McCrae J, Whitten-Shurney W, Thomas R, Bond S 2001. Characterization of pica prevalence among patients with sickle cell disease. *Arch Pediatr Adolesc Med* 155(11):1243–1247.

Karimi MR, Kadivar R, Yarmohammadi H 2002. Assessment of the prevalence of iron deficiency anemia, by serum ferritin, in pregnant women of Southern Iran. *Med Sci Monit* 8:CR448-492.

Katz JM. Poor Haitians resort to eating dirt. National Geographic News. (Accessed 03-21-2017). Available at: http://news.nationalgeographic.com/news/2008/01/080130/AP-haiti-eaten

Kawai K, Saathoff E, Antelman G, Msamanga G, Fawzi WW 2009. Geophagy (soil-eating) in relation to anemia and helminth infection among HIV-infected pregnant women in Tanzania. *Am J Trop Med Hyg* 80(1):36–43.

Khoushabi F, Ahmadi P, Shadan MR, Heydari A, Miri M, Jamnejad M 2014. Pica practices among pregnant women are associated with lower hemoglobin levels and pregnancy outcome. *Open J Obstet Gynecol* 4(11):7 pages.

Knishinsky R 1998. *The Benefits of Clay*. Healing Art Press, Rochester, Vermont.

Lopez LB, Ortega Soler CR, de Portela ML 2004. Pica during pregnancy: A frequently underestimated problem. *Arch Latinoam Nutr* 54(1):17–24.

Luoba AI, Geissler PW, Estambale B, Ouma JH, Magnussen P, Alusala D, Ayah R, Mwaniki D, Friis H 2004. Geophagy among pregnant and lactating women in Bondo District, western Kenya. *Trans R Soc Trop Med Hyg* 98(12):734–741.

Marchi M, Cohen P 1990. Early childhood eating behaviors and adolescent eating disorders. *J Am Acad Child Adolesc Psychiatry* 29(1):112–117.

Mawathe A 2008. *Why Kenyan Women Crave Stones.* British Broadcasting Corporation. Available at: http://news.bbc.co.uk/2/hi/7596067.stm

McAlpine C, Singh NN 1986. Pica in institutionalized mentally retarded persons. *J Ment Defic Res* 30(2):171–178.

McLoughlin IJ 1987. The picas. *Br J Hosp Med* 37: 286–90.

Nchito M, Geissler PW, Mubila L, Friss H, Olsen A 2004. Effects of iron and multi-micronutrient supplementation on geophagy: A two-by-two factorial study among Zambian schoolchildren in Lusaka. *Trans R Soc Trop Med Hyg* 98(4):218–227.

Ngole VM, Ekosse GE, de Jager L, Songca SP 2010. Physicochemical characteristics of geophagic clayey soils from South Africa and Swaziland. *Afr J Biotechnol* 9(36):5929–5937.

Ngozi PO 2008. Pica practices of pregnant women in Nairobi, Kenya. *East Afr Med J* 85(2):72–79.

Njiru H, Elchalal U, Paltiel O 2011. Geophagy during pregnancy in Africa: A literature review. *Obstet Gynecol Surv* 66(7):452–459.

Nyaruhucha CN 2009. Food cravings, aversions and pica among pregnant women in Dar es Salaam, Tanzania. *Tanzan J Health* 11(1):29–34.

Rainville AJ 1998. Pica practices of pregnant women are associated with lower maternal hemoglobin level at delivery. *J Am Diet Assoc* 98(3):293–296.

Roselle HA 1970. Association of laundry starch and clay ingestion with anaemia in New York City. *Arab Intern Med* 125:57–61.

Saathoff E, Olsen A, Kvalsvig JD, Geissler PW 2002. Geophagy and its association with geohelminth infection in rural schoolchildren from northern KwaZuluNatal, South Africa. *Trans R Soc Trop Med Hyg* 96(5):485–490.

Saunders C, Padilha PC, Della LB 2009. Pica: epidemiology and association with pregnancy complications [in Portuguese]. *Rev Bras Ginecol Obstet* 31:440–446.

Schmidt B, Ayer A (editors) 2009. Dirt Poor Haitians Eat Mud Cookies to Survive. Huffington Post. Available at: http://www.huffingtonpost. com/2009/02/19/dirt-poor-haitians-eat-mu_n_168339.html

Shinondo C, Mwikuma G 2009. Geophagy as a risk factor for helminth infections in pregnant women in Lusaka, Zambia. *Med J Zambia* 35:48–52.

Shivoga WA, Moturi WN 2009. Geophagia as a risk factor for diarrhoea. *J Infect Dev Ctries* 3(2):94–98.

Simpson E, Mull J, Longley E, East J 2000. Pica during pregnancy in low-income women born in Mexico. *West J Med* 173:20–24.

The Hindu 2015. A Secret Addiction in Old Hyderabad. Available at: https://www.thehindu.com/features/magazine/nikhila-henry-on-the-stoneeaters-of-hyderabad/article7641379.ece

Thompson LC 2009. *William Scott Ament and the Boxer Rebellion.* Jefferson, NC: McFarland. p. 21.

Twenefour D 1999. A study of clay ingestion among lactating and pregnant women in the greater Accra region and associated motives and effects. Bsc. Dissertation submitted to the Department of Nutrition and Food Science, University of Ghana, Legon.

Vermeer DE 1966. Geophagy among the Tiv of Nigeria. *Ann Assoc Am Geogr* 56(2):197–204.

Vermeer DE, Frate DA 1979. Geophagia in rural Mississippi: Environmental and cultural contexts and nutritional implications. *Am J Clin Nutr* 32:2129–2135.

Walker ARP, Walker BF, Sookaria F, Canan RJ 1997. Pica. *J R Soc Health* 1147(5):280–284.

Wayne F 2004. *Dixie Forgotten People: The Poor Whites.* Indiana University Press, p. 40.

Wikipedia, The Free Encyclopedia 2017a. Geophagy. Available at: https:// en.wikipedia.org/wiki/Geophagia#cite_note-12

Wikipedia, The Free Encyclopedia 2017b. The Northern Chinese Famine of 1876–79. Available at: https://en.wikipedia.org/wiki/Northern_ Chinese_Famine_of_1876%E2%80%9379

Woywodt A, Kiss A 2002. Geophagia: The history of earth-eating. *J R Soc Med* 95:143–146.

Young SL, Khalfan SS, Farag TH, Kavle JA, Ali SM, Hajji H, Rasmussen KM, Pelto GH, Tielsch JM, Stoltzfus RJ 2010. Association of pica with anemia and gastrointestinal distress among pregnant women in Zanzibar, Tanzania. *Am J Trop Med Hyg* 83(1):144–151.

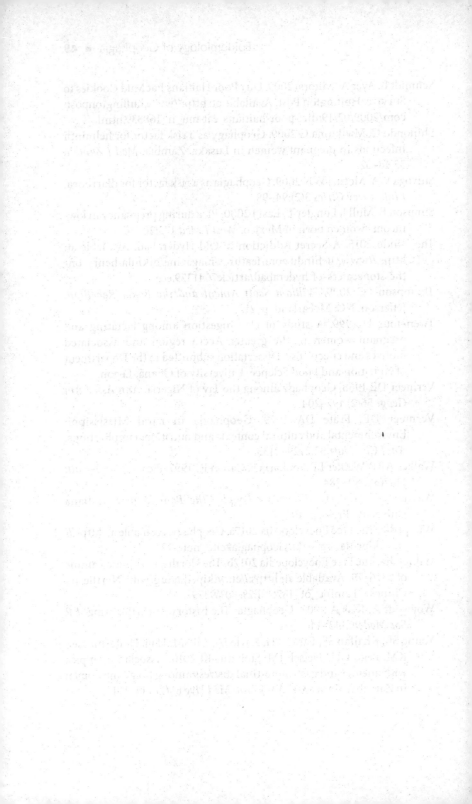

CHAPTER 4

Etiology of Geophagia

4.1 INTRODUCTION

It is not an exaggeration to say that the habit of geophagia coincides with the history of mankind. It has worldwide prevalence and longstanding persistence across several human generations. The habit of geophagia has been described by many writers in their manuscripts. Nevertheless, these references are highly fragmented and deliver abstruse illustrations concerning the age, gender, and occupation of individuals eating non-foods. Additionally, the descriptions in ancient texts about the type and quantity of ingested clay are insufficient to draw fruitful conclusions. Moreover, depictions of geophagia in the literature are supplemented with insufficient and dissenting evidence about the predisposing factors for geophagia and marked with disagreement among various thinkers about uniform criteria for the diagnosis of geophagia and its effects on human body tissues. The ancient postulations about geophagia are silent concerning universally acceptable interventional measures to terminate the habit of geophagia.

Plausible causative factors that have been put forward by various thinkers are described in the present section of this book.

4.2 MICRONUTRIENT DEFICIENCY

Micronutrients are elements that are required by organisms in trace amounts essential to sustain normal growth and development (UNICEF 2017; WHO and FAO 2004). In the human body, the daily requirement of micronutrients is less than 100 mg (Gernand et al. 2016). Micronutrients include iron, iodine, zinc, selenium, magnesium, manganese, and vitamins (USDA 2017).

Micronutrients are wonder elements that are essential for biosynthesis of hormones, enzymes, macromolecules, and nucleic acids in the bodies of organisms (WHO 2017a).

The micronutrient deficiency hypothesis states, "Inadequacy of micronutrients is the prime etiological factor for the arousal of physiological need that intensely motivates affected individuals to fulfill micronutrient deficiency by adapting an aberrant behavior related to eating of soil, clay, or any other earth-related non-food substances."

A conceptual framework linking micronutrient deficiency and clay eating has been suggested by the author that encompasses five elements.

1. *Increased Physiological Need for Micronutrients*: Pregnancy is a physiological period of life for women in the reproductive age group. It is characterized by vast physiological and metabolic changes in a woman's body (Mridula et al. 2003). The most significant change is the increase in plasma volume (Ladipo 2000), which is further associated with a decrease in the quantity of micronutrients and albumin in plasma (Cross et al. 1995). The deficiency of micronutrients in pregnant

women is further aggravated in cases where dietary intake is poor, especially in poor populations in remote places, villages, the tribal belt, and nomadic people residing in developing and developed countries as in Figure 4.1 (Ladipo 2000; Black 2001).

According to Darnton-Hill and Mkparu (2015), the requirement for micronutrients is increased in pregnancy. Micronutrients are used to fulfill the elevated metabolic

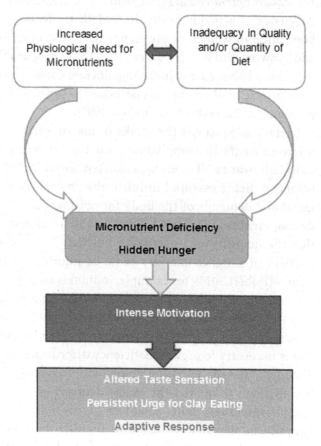

FIGURE 4.1 Conceptual framework of micronutrient deficiency hypothesis.

demands of the body in pregnant women and are essential to fulfilling the nutritional requirements of the growing fetus.

According to IFPRI (2014), it was estimated that around 2 billion people, including pregnant women and preschool children, were suffering from acute deficiency of micronutrients.

2. *Inadequate Quantity and Poor Quality of Diet*: Micronutrient deficiency is a major health hazard that affects a large population of women in pregnancy (Gernand et al. 2016) and growing children (Bhan et al. 2001). It is desirable to consume a balanced diet including different edibles selected from diverse food groups. It is necessary to supply essential nutrients for the body (Wasantwisut 1997).

Dietary adequacy is the intake of macronutrients and micronutrients in compliance with the recommended daily allowance (Dhonukshe-Rutten et al. 2013). A balanced diet is essential to fulfill the physiological and metabolic demands of the body for optimal growth and development as in Figure 4.1 (Gupta 2015). It is noteworthy that the quantity of a particular nutrient is variable. A nutrient in a higher quantity could be injurious to body tissues (Robert 2013); for example, sodium is an important mineral of extracellular fluid and its intake exceeding the recommended daily allowance could predispose a person to hypertension. Gupta (2015) suggested that adequacy of diet is necessary to prevent deficiency disorders, systemic disorders, and malnutrition among children and adults. It is difficult to predict the exact adequacy of a diet for every individual (NRC 1986). Moreover, inadequate quantity in the diet is unable to furnish the requisite calories and minerals to the human body. Therefore, inadequacy of diet is responsible for deficiency of calories and micronutrients.

Further, adequacy of food quality is another important paradigm to prevent deficiency of micronutrients in the body. Food quality is the characteristics of the food that are agreeable to consumers and enhance the palatability of food (USDA and NIFA 2019).

According to FAO (2005), food quality represents the texture and nutritional value of food. It depends on selection of food items from particular food groups, such as the selection of protein from animal sources, which provides a better quality of protein in comparison to plant sources; according to Vliet et al. (2015), plant-source proteins have less digestibility than animal-source proteins. The authors found that intake of proteins like wheat and soy from plants provided less muscle protein synthetic response than proteins from animals. Therefore, poor food quality is the cause of deficiency of calories and essential minerals in the body.

3. *Micronutrient Deficiency or Hidden Hunger*: Poverty leading to insufficient procurement of food for the family (Zalilah and Ang 2001; Zalilah and Tham 2002), natural calamity (Artur and Hilhorst 2014), state policy resulting in inadequate food storage (FAO 2019) for the population, and famine are the major factors that are responsible for starvation and hidden hunger. According to WHO (2017), hidden hunger is the consequence of prolonged intake of a low-quality diet (Thompson and Amoroso 2014), which is detrimental to the growth and development of body. The World Health Organization (2017) estimated that about 2 billion people suffer from micronutrient deficiency. The condition was worse among pregnant women and preschool children owing to an increase in the physiological demand for micronutrients in the body during pregnancy and lactation in women and in formative age groups in children as in Figure 4.1 (Katz 2008; Christian 2010).

> Consequently, mineral deficiency in the body of an individual is a strong physiological drive and therefore has been postulated as the key functional drive for geophagia among pregnant women and preschool children. (Castro and Boyd-Orr, 1952)

4. *Motivation and Urge for Clay Eating*: According to Maslow's hierarchy of needs, motivation is necessary to achieve one's needs in order to have a healthy body and mind. The theory postulates five levels of human needs, which are called the hierarchy of needs.

According to the theory, it is essential to fulfill one's basic needs like hunger, sex, and thirst, which are represented by the lowest level of the five-level model of needs (Maslow 1943). This determines a person's behavior. It is necessary for the survival of the human race. Inability to achieve any one of the basic needs strongly motivates and molds the behavior of a person for the accomplishment of the need.

> It is hypothesized that nutritional deficiency in preschool children and pregnant women is the strong motivational force that drives them to adapt to indiscriminate eating patterns.

> The reward system is the assembly of neuronal structures in the brain that are implicated in reward behavior that is composed of motivation, incessant desire, strong craving, and reward (Schultz 2015). This behavior is also associated with positive reinforcement, conditioning, and pleasure-seeking motive or to achieve a state of euphoria (Berridge and Kringelbach 2015).

Dopaminergic pathways are the neuronal networks that connect one portion of brain with another. They are composed of axons of dopaminergic neurons in the brain. There are three main types of dopaminergic pathways: nigrostriatal, mesolimbic, and mesocortical pathways. The mesolimbic pathway is primarily implicated in reward behavior. The cell bodies of the mesolimbic pathway are located in the ventral tegmental area at the floor of the midbrain (Malenka et al. 2009). The axons descend from the ventral tegmental area to the ventral corpus striatum, which is located in the forebrain. The ventral corpus striatum is the chief component of the reward system of the brain (Yager et al. 2015). It is composed of the nucleus accumbens and olfactory tubercle (Ferré et al. 2010; Taylor et al. 2013).

Dopamine is discharged from dopamine neurons, and it binds to dopamine receptors D1 and D2 in the brain (Tritsch and Sabatini 2012). Dopamine is the key neurotransmitter responsible for reward behavior (Calabresi et al. 2014), reinforcing behavior, conditioning, and memory.

The dopaminergic system is also incriminated in the pathogenesis of diseases like depression, schizophrenia, Huntington disease, Parkinson disease, and addiction to chemicals (Kravitz et al. 2010; Hyun and Antonio 2012).

Moreover, aberrant behavior like geophagia could be related to decreased dopaminergic activity in the brain. A study was conducted by Youdim et al. (1983) on rats wherein iron deficiency was induced. Youdim et al. (1983) observed that iron deficiency was responsible for a decrease in dopamine to dopamine receptor binding sites in the brains of the experimental rats. This activity materialized into a corresponding reduction in dopaminergic activity in the brain (Youdim et al. 1983). The authors suggested that it could lead to diminished dopaminergic activity in the brain of experimental rats. Further, Youdim et al. (1983) mentioned that the findings in dopaminergic activity in experimental rats with induced iron deficiency were similar to observations in animal models that were treated with psychotropic drugs.

Youdim et al. (1983) pointed out that dietary iron deficiency could cause impairment in the synthesis of protein in the brain. It is the basis of a reduction in the number of dopamine receptors and dopaminergic activity that in turn could predispose one to altered behavior and psychiatric disorders in children with a nutritional iron deficit (Youdim et al. 1983, 1984).

Further, Beard et al. (1994), Bianco et al. (2008), and Unger et al. (2014) posited that dietary iron deficiency could impair dopaminergic neurotransmission, which could lead to reduced functioning of dopamine transporters and dopamine receptor D2 in the ventral corpus striatum.

Conclusion

Therefore, it is speculated that diminished dopaminergic activity in the brain is manifested as altered eating behavior.

Dopamine has an important role in motivation, behavior reinforcement, learning, distinguishing between good and bad things, and performing good things to achieve pleasure and avoid pain (Montague et al. 1996).

According to Schultz (1998), dopaminergic neurons in the ventral tegmental area, nucleus accumbens in the midbrain, are actively responsible for reward and reinforcing behavior. A stimulus like drinking water and palatable food elicits high dopaminergic activity in the brain, and the phenomenon is called phasic bursts in the midbrain. The author postulated that neurons show phases of activation and depression following stimuli that ensure reward.

Therefore, appetite motivates an individual to hunt for and procure food and achieve satiety, a sense of reward. Hence, this behavior becomes reinforced. During a deficiency of micronutrients in body, which is also called hidden hunger, the individual is apparently not hungry, but the bioavailability of minerals like iron, calcium, and zinc is compromised in the body.

Hidden hunger motivates an individual voraciously to fulfill the physiological need for minerals. The individual compulsively engages in the eating of clay, soil, or plaster in order to achieve a reward or sense of satiety. Later on, altered eating behavior becomes conditioned. It might be an adaptive response to micronutrient deficiency.

A deficiency of vitamin A and trace minerals like iron and iodine in the body is mainly responsible for hidden hunger (UNICEF 2017).

It might be concluded that nutritional iron deficiency and the resulting iron deficit in the brain might be responsible for decreased protein synthesis and hence a reduction in the number of dopaminergic receptors. The condition is linked to diminished dopaminergic activity in the midbrain. Otherwise, dopamine is a neurotransmitter that is necessary for reward-expecting behavior, motivation, learning, and behavior reinforcement.

Altered eating behavior might be linked to diminished dopaminergic activity. Additional research is warranted to reach a final conclusion.

4.2.1 Descriptive Evidence

A study by Gregory (1995) described that dietary iron intake among preschool children with geophagia was low. Another study by James (1989) observed that preschool children suffered from iron deficiency and anemia.

The active growth period among preschool children has a high physiological demand for minerals. This becomes a strong motivation for a few predisposed children to indulge in the practice of clay eating (Singhi et al. 2003).

A study by Johnson (1990) was conducted in Western countries among patients who were addicted to the habit of pica. Johnson (1990) reported the highest prevalence of iron deficiency in patients with a pica habit, which in turn could be associated with iron-deficiency anemia or not. Moreover, Johnson (1990) asserted that the habit of pica was observed in around 50% of patients with an iron deficiency.

Sugita (2001) commented that pica consumers have the highest prevalence of deficiency of micronutrients like iron, calcium, and zinc in the body.

Crosby (1976) was a strong proponent of the functional hypothesis of geophagia and stated that pica is the clinical manifestation of an iron deficiency in the body of an individual and is directly related to reduction in total body iron stores. Additionally, Crosby (1976) posited that geophagia is not the direct outcome of anemia. Further, the author stated that pica is highly uncommon in anemia other than iron-deficiency anemia. Moreover, Crosby (1976) posited that pica is terminated after iron replacement is instituted.

Johnson (1990) could not put forward an explanation for a relation between iron deficiency in the body and an abnormal eating tendency. The author suggested that iron is an important constituent of digestive enzymes, and a reduced iron store might be implicated in abnormal behavior to fulfill iron needs through delinquent eating behavior.

Again, pica is also associated with a deficiency of zinc in the body, apart from iron deficiency. Therefore, absolute iron deficiency is not the cause of geophagia.

Cavdar et al. (1983) and Zedlitz (2010) have stated their views that geophagia is a reactive response to physiological demands during pregnancy, lactation, and childhood, wherein the requirement for micronutrients is higher.

4.2.2 Clinical Trials

A case was reported by Barton et al. (2016) in which the patient was a woman in the middle age group and a resident of Mumbai, India. The patient had a strong desire to eat uncooked basmati rice. Barton et al. (2016) found that the patient suffered from fatigue, loss of hair, and pallor. The authors observed microcytic anemia and deficiency of iron after laboratory investigation. Barton et al. (2016) managed the patient with an intravenous administration of iron. It was reported by the authors that the habit of pica was discontinued after the initial dose of iron.

A similar case of eating uncooked rice was reported by Barton et al. (2016). The patient was from Karachi, Pakistan, and was a middle-aged woman. She was lethargic, with defective growth of nails, and had a feeling of giddiness, as observed by the authors. After examination, Barton et al. (2016) found that the patient suffered from pallor and had microcytic anemia. She was treated by the authors through administration of iron supplements, and she recovered from the habit of pica successfully (Barton et al. 2016).

Additional clinical evidence was provided by Rwegerera et al. (2015). The patient was a primary school–going boy. Rwegerera et al. (2015) narrated symptoms of headache, giddiness, and palpitation in the boy. He belonged to a poor family. Rwegerera et al. (2015) observed a history of clay eating, severe anemia, and poor intake of food for the past 2 years. After laboratory investigation, Rwegerera et al. (2015) noted that the boy's hemoglobin level was 2.9 g% and total iron was 13.3 mmol/L.

Rwegerera et al. (2015) recommended hospitalization; the boy underwent a transfusion of blood and was administered iron supplements. The boy dropped the habit of clay eating after treatment for the next 6 months.

4.2.3 Evidence against Micronutrient Deficiency

Ingestion of clay and soil damage the mucosa of the alimentary canal. This leads to inflammation of the mucosa, which impairs its absorptive capability; this condition is called environmental enteropathy (Campbell et al. 2003a,b). This hypothesis states that geophagia is the cause of malabsorption syndrome and mineral deficiency among children.

A contrasting view was put forward by Johns and Duquette (1991), Horner et al. (1991), and Hooda et al. (2002). According to them, ingestion of clay and other constituents of soil enter the gut and interfere with the absorption of dietary micronutrients by chelating them. Hence, absorption of micronutrients like iron and zinc is obstructed, which in turn manifests as mineral deficiency.

Arcasoy et al. (1978) studied iron absorption between two groups of children. The authors observed that iron absorption was slower among children who practiced geophagia in contrast to children in the control group.

Another case of geophagia was reported by Cavdar et al. (1983) among Turkish children and women who resided in villages. These individuals practiced clay eating. Children and women presented symptoms of growth retardation and delayed puberty. Cavdar et al. (1983) estimated serum concentration of zinc and iron and found decreased concentrations of both iron and zinc in the sera of children and women.

Cavdar et al. (1983) conducted oral absorption tests of zinc and iron in the presence of clay and without its presence. It was observed by the authors that clay interfered in the absorption of iron and zinc, and the authors postulated that Turkish clay inhibits absorption of iron and zinc, resulting in a deficiency disorder with myriad manifestations.

4.2.4 Critical Analysis

The micronutrient deficiency hypothesis incorporates two contrasting viewpoints about the etiopathogenesis of geophagy.

- The studies conducted by Castro and Boyd-Orr (1952), Crosby (1976), Johnson (1990), Gregory (1995), and Singhi et al. (2003) suggest that geophagia is the effect of a deficiency of micronutrients in the body of a patient that drives a strong urge to fulfill the deficiency through altered eating behavior.

- Moreover, Arcasoy et al. (1978), Horner et al. (1991), Johns and Duquette (1991), Hooda et al. (2002), and Campbell et al. (2003) conversely stated that geophagia is the cause of inflammation of the gut mucosa. Moreover, geophagia predisposes one to decreased solubility of iron and other minerals in the lumen of the small intestine, which leads to diminished absorption of dietary minerals. Therefore, geophagia is the cause of mineral deficiency in the body.

- It is highly disputative to reach a conclusion on the etiology of geophagia. Furthermore, it could be inferred that geophagia might start due to mineral deficiency, which later on exaggerates mineral deficiency through multiple mechanisms; hence, acute mineral deficiency might reinforce the behavior of the individual (Lacey 1990; Brand et al. 2009a).

4.3 PSYCHOLOGICAL STRESS

This hypothesis asserts that pica is a psychopathological disorder that arises in response to either external or internal psychological stress stimuli.

Psychological stress is a state of tension that arises owing to an imbalance between extraordinary demands and the ability of an individual to cope with those demands. It is manifested in terms of physiological and emotional disturbances in an individual upon anticipating a situation where the expectations surpass the coping strategies.

Psychological stress can be defined in terms of stimulus as an external (environmental) event, which can trigger a cascade of physiological reactions in the human body.

Psychological stress can also be defined in terms of response, as the complex physiological reactions of the body in response to hostile stimuli.

Hans Selye (1956) defined stress as the non-specific response of the individual's body to any external stimulus. The author posited that stress can be positive when the stimulus brings about an improvement in the performance or productivity of an individual. Such a stress is called eustress.

Furthermore, Selye (1956) suggested that stress can be negative when the stimulus brings about a decline in either performance or productivity or creates psychological problems. Such a stress is called distress.

4.3.1 Descriptive Evidence in Favor of the Hypothesis

Blinder et al. (1988) observed the parent-child relationship to comment on the cause of the geophagia habit in children. They reported mal-aligned parent-child relations as the etiological basis of geophagia in children. Blinder et al. (1988) described emotionally deprived children as being more susceptible to the habits of geophagia and pica.

Goldstein (1998) reported an female African American patient of 33 years of age who had the habit of pica. Goldstein (1998) described that the woman had suffered loss and embarrassment in her life, and explained that the practice of pica in the woman was a consolation for the psychological trauma she had suffered in the past.

Edwards et al. (1994) and Cooskey (1995) reported a strong relation between pica and psychological stress among pregnant women. The authors described how the eating of ice cubes by pregnant women helped to relive stress. Rose et al. (2000) posited that pagophagia was linked to a narrow social support system and shrunken social lineage. The author described pagophagia as a compensatory mechanism for poor social associations that helped relive stress.

Geophagia and pica among adults is a result of mental retardation and psychiatric disorders (Bhatia and Gupta 2009). According to Hunter (2004), the American Dietetic Association considers geophagia a behavioral disorder. Persons with developmental disabilities are more inclined to the habits of pica and geophagia.

Geophagia is a perverted dietary behavior and requires psychoanalysis and psychotherapy to control it (APA 2011).

A descriptive study was conducted by Singhi et al. (1981) on a total of 100 children to assess the effect of psychological stress on the habit of geophagia. The authors assigned 50 children with iron deficiency and the habit of geophagia to one group, whereas the other assigned group had another 50 children who were anemic (Singhi et al. 1981), but did not have the habit of geophagia. It was observed by Singhi et al. (1981) that children with the habit of geophagia suffered from higher levels of stress in comparison to the group of children without the habit of geophagia. Singhi et al. (1981) posited that divorce of parents, deprivation of parental care, poor family structure, child abuse, and insufficient parental care of children were the predisposing factors for stress and were intimately related to the habit of geophagia among children.

Another study was conducted by Bithoney et al. (1985) in preschool children that was related to the effects of family stress on the habit of geophagia. The authors prepared an interview schedule covering factors like family stress, family structure, child temperament, social responsiveness of the child, and parental attitude as representative of family stress. The authors interviewed hospitalized children and their parents. Overall, it was concluded by Bithoney et al. (1985) that the practice of geophagia was associated with family stress.

Edwards et al. (1994) asserted that the habit of pagophagia ("pagos" means frost) is a reinforcement behavior that is intended to cope with psychological stress. Unhealthy social interaction, according to Edwards et al. (1994), is the cause of stress that could predispose one to the habit of pagophagia.

According to the APA (2011), in Western psychology, general pica behavior is considered a psychopathology requiring intervention. Pica is typically associated with high levels of stress, anxiety, depression, and developmental disorders (Danford et al. 1982; Stiegler 2005; Stroman et al. 2011). Cravings for substances, in some instances, are comparable to those for opium and alcohol, with consumption alleviating psychological discomfort (Edwards et al. 1994, Young 2011).

4.4 HUNGER HYPOTHESIS

This hypothesis describes the habit of geophagia on the basis of the hunger drive in humans. Poverty, hunger, and starvation are the motivational forces to eat earth substances like clay, soil, and kaolin in the absence of adequate food sources in order to achieve a sense of satiety.

Pica is frequently practiced in regions experiencing starvation and poverty, leading to intake of non-foods to reduce hunger (Hawass et al. 1987).

4.4.1 Descriptive Evidence in Favor

Young (2010) differentiated between a feeling of hunger and an intense urge for earth eating and posited that persons have been observed eating clay even after having had a full meal. Further, a proponent of the hunger hypothesis (Bourne 2008) mentioned that non-food substances could relieve hunger pangs. According to this theory, some individuals are addicted to amylophagia (starch eating), where a person consumes lot of starch to achieve satiety that could provide calories to body.

Therefore, the hunger hypothesis requires further research to answer the pathogenesis of geophagia.

According to a blog (Chokhi Dhani 2014), the battle of Haldighati forced Maharana Pratap and his family members to take shelter in a forest. The royal family had to feed upon preparations made from grass stems.

Another explanation of geophagia on the basis of the hunger hypothesis was provided by Bateson and Lebroy (1978) in their work on Aboriginals who practiced geophagia. The authors posited that clay consumption was neither attributed to pregnancy nor iron-deficiency anemia or perverted appetite. Possibly, according to the authors, the habit of geophagia was attributed to hunger, which reinforced their behavior to seek pleasure through clay consumption.

4.4.2 Critical Analysis of Hypothesis

On the basis of the above-cited evidence, it can be assumed that eating of non-food items becomes essential in hunger for survival. Possible assertions can be put forward as follows:

- Individuals consume non-food items in the absence of food scarcity.

- Individuals practice geophagia (pica) to satisfy hunger.

- Geophagia (pica) is practiced by individuals voluntarily in food scarcity conditions; nevertheless, the practice is discontinued after the availability of foods increases.

- In food scarcity, whatever is available, food or non-food, becomes the choice of affected individuals.

According to Corbett (1988), Butterley and Sheperd (2010), and Hadley and Crooks (2012), food insecurity motivates people to search for fodder that is widespread in the region and not eaten during periods of food sufficiency. The fodder fulfills the necessity of foods in adverse conditions.

According to author (Ray 2002), spiders fried are eaten in regions of Cambodia. According to Corbett (1988), Moser (1996), and Hadley and Crooks (2012), a food scarcity–afflicted population searches for foods that might be less nutritious, easily available, and cheaper, or for non-nutritious foods in place of vitamin-rich foods.

According to Corbett (1988) and Shipton (1990), food-insecure populations are compelled to consume proscribed foods, which can be termed famine foods. This practice is prevalent in times of food adversity.

According to Morton (1953), throughout the Battle of Bataan, in the Philippines, the population consumed meat of dogs, monkeys, and monitor lizards because of the reduced supply of food items in World War II.

The origin of this dietary habit is unclear; however, it is posited that the habit of eating stigmatized food might have originated during times of food scarcity in the rule of the Khmer Rouge.

According to Yves and Dechassa (2000), the buds and berries of the flower *Capparis spinosa* are considered famine foods in the drought-hit areas of southern Ethiopia.

4.5 CULTURE HYPOTHESIS

According to the Cambridge English Dictionary, culture is the lifestyle adopted by a localized group of people, particularly the customs and beliefs at a specific point in time (CED 2017).

A famous anthropologist, Taylor, said that culture is a complex entity that encompasses knowledge, law, customs, beliefs, and any additional habit that is learned by an individual in a society.

According to Paul et al. (2015), culture is a social trait that underlines certain habits, practices, and discourses, which becomes the matrix for coherence and incoherence of social life over time.

Geophagia in certain societies of world still persists as a culture. The practice has its roots in the traditions, rituals, and religion of that society. Culture-motivated geophagia exhibits differences in comparison to geophagia practiced by children in the formative years of life and mentally challenged individuals. Culture-associated geophagia involves intentional, but nonetheless irresistible, eating of clay and kaolin that might be procured from a commercial market. Moreover, children 2–3 years of age and mentally disturbed persons are ignorant about the substances that are put in the mouth.

Frate (1984) reported in his work that the belief was deeply instilled in the mind of people concerning the medicinal properties of clay. Frate (1984) mentioned the term "terra sigilata," or "sealed earth," in his work and described its prevalence among Greeks to cure various ailments in 40 BC. Further, Frate (1984) described how clay was extracted by the priests from specified areas of Lemnos (an island in Greece) to obtain the medicinal properties of the clay. Frate (1984) mentioned certain rituals that were essential to purify clay before its use. With the passage of time, clay eating became a habit among selected people.

Indigenous peoples of the Unites States have been described as consuming soil. Hunter (1973) stated that a culture of soil eating in South America was transmitted from West African populations during slavery. Why slaves indulged in the practice of soil eating has not been understood by thinkers. One possibility is intentionally acquiring sickness by consuming soil (Hunter 1973).

Conversely, soil eating was considered distasteful by Americans due to its harmful effects. Primarily, it was a contentious source of intestinal parasites.

Lacey (1990) strongly argued that, according to the theory of causation of geophagia, a single cause is considered the etiopathogenesis of geophagia and that this is highly inappropriate, as it is multifactorial in pathogenesis. Lacey (1990) stated that ethnicity or culture was ignored while framing the definition and etiology of geophagia. Lacey (1990) further explained that geophagia is common in West African populations, who have a natural inclination to consume clay and kaolin. Lacey (1990) posited that premeditated eating of clay in West Africans was intended to render themselves ill intentionally. This behavior could make them physically unfit for slavery and save them from the clutches of kings. The habit of clay eating was passed from one generation to another and, with the passage of time, became a cultural trait (Lacey 1990).

4.5.1 Descriptive Evidence in Favor of Culture Hypothesis

In countries with hot climates, it is a common practice to eat clay among pregnant women and children, especially among the inhabitants of rural areas and slums. This habit is acquired, practiced, and deeply rooted in the minds of members of society. According to Abrahams and Parsons (1996), clay and other forms of pica are commercialized for common intake in formulations like tablets. In Cameroon, kaolin is available in markets for geophagia material and may be flavored with black pepper and cardamom (BBC News 2016). In Haiti, biscuits are prepared by mixing clay, salt, and butter to be available for human use in geophagia (Benno and Ara 2009). In rural areas of Mississippi, baked and processed dirt and clay consumption has been a common practice by poor populations of whites and blacks for many generations.

It is hard to decipher the precise reason for the rise of geophagia in a society as a culture-bound phenomenon. According to Gelfand (1945), it was believed by local populations that soil has the potential to support fertility among women and lessen the complications that follow delivery. These beliefs were practiced through generations even without any scientific evidence. According to Geissler (2000), soil eating is a custom in Luoland in Western Kenya among primary school children. Adolescent children and women consume clay. In African countries, earth eating by females represents their feminine identity (Vermeer 1966), while children's liking or disliking eating earth reveals their developing gender (Geissler 2000). Earth represents a feminine symbol and the power of fertility. Earth is eaten by groups of women of reproductive age and is hidden from male members of society. Therefore, earth eating in most African societies is considered a sacred union with forces of reproduction and is a deep-seated cultural practice (Geissler 2000). The Chagga community commonly practices geophagia. The Chagga community is one of the largest ethnic groups in Tanzania. The Chagga community relates the fertility of women to the fertility of soil. According to Moore and Puritt (1977), Chagga women eat clay, kaolin, and mud in the belief that it will increase their fertility. It has become an acquired trait in Chagga women. Soil eating is a cultural practice among regional populations throughout the world, and it has a highly complex etiology of origin; nevertheless, cultural geophagia revolves around a deeply engraved tradition of continuity from one generation to the next over time.

According to Grigsby et al. (1999), geophagia is a worldwide practice that has been documented by various workers across the world. However, intake of kaolin is less common than eating soil. Kaolin is white clay, and its eating has been widely practiced, according to Grigsby et al. (1999), among the inhabitants of the Piedmont plateau in central Georgia. Grigsby et al. (1999) collected information about the habit through interaction with local physicians and conducting interviews with the affected population. Grigsby et al. (1999) asserted that kaolin eating among the population in the Piedmont plateau is culture bound and might be unassociated with any psychiatric disorder. This culture-bound issue can be defined according to the DSM-IV (APA 1994) as a repetitive and deviant eating behavior that is locality centered, and its linkage to a category in the DSM-IV is either established or remains dissociated.

According to Johns (1990), indigenous populations practiced the use of clay during the preparation of foods. According to Johns (1990), ingredients of clay that consisted of components of rock, silica, and magnesium salts feasibly adsorbed harmful contaminants that were present in foods.

The use of natural clay has been a custom to alleviate gastrointestinal disturbances like diarrhea and hyperacidity and as a detoxification agent. Carretero (2002) analyzed the native clay of a quarry in Bingerville using modern instrumentation techniques. Carretero (2002) found that a clay mineral called kaolinite was the predominant constituent of clay and described the presence of minerals like copper, zinc, cobalt, and molybdenum, which could be beneficial to humans, and the occurrence of a very low amount of heavy metals like lead and cadmium that are toxic to humans.

According to Wiley and Solomon (1998), eating clay was a cultural practice among sub-Saharan Africans that was transferred to their progeny. The origin of geophagia could be traced to the positive effects of clays that were consumed during pregnancy by women. Wiley and Solomon (1998) argued for the antiemetic effects of clays in the first trimester of pregnancy. Further, the authors posited that ingested clays could have the property of supplementing calcium in the second trimester of pregnancy. A plausible explanation for eating clay by the sub-Saharan African population as a culture could be the awareness of the medicinal properties of clays that their ancestors possessed and was passed to the coming generations through the cultural practice of geophagia. The timing of eating clays by pregnant women coincided with the onset of symptoms of nausea, vomiting, and gastric disturbances in the first and second trimesters of pregnancy. According to Wiley and Solomon (1998), the sites of procuring clays were predetermined; nevertheless, the quantity and timing of clay consumption could vary in different tribal populations. Wiley and Solomon (1998) provided important information regarding the trade of clays through an established network of clay traders who had their approach in urban areas.

According to Wiley and Solomon (1998), clays with the aforementioned medicinal properties were obtained from the mounds of termites. Debatably, the accumulation of minerals like phosphorus, calcium, iron, and potassium has been documented in termite mounds by another researcher (Van Huis 1996). Wiley and Solomon (1998) concluded cultural geophagia among the sub-Saharan African population existed and termed this practice as predating *Homo sapiens*.

The consumption of soils from termite mounds had also been reported by Hunter (1984), and it was practiced as a part of culture by pregnant women in Africa. Hunter (1984) stated that the soils could be dried and baked over the fire before their use by individuals. According to Njiru et al. (2011), consumption of termite soils by African women was attributed to strong urges that developed in pregnancy. Njiru et al. (2011) collected information from sources that mentioned the use of termite soils to fulfill the requirement of iron in pregnancy. This fact was further confirmed by the work of Luoba et al. (2004) with pregnant and lactating women in Western Kenya who practiced geophagia. Luoba et al. (2004) reported a prevalence of 65% of geophagia among pregnant women. The important sources of soils, as reported by the authors, were soft stones, known as odowa, and termite mounds.

Van Huis (1996) documented in his work the availability of 14% of dietary iron that was essentially recommended during pregnancy.

Regarding the time period of clay consumption in pregnancy, Hunter (1984) mentioned that clays were consumed in the first and second trimesters of pregnancy and, in some cases, they were eaten over all periods of pregnancy. Hunter (1984) further documented the nature of clays eaten by women. More often, clays like kaolin and montmorillonite (soft clay with medicinal properties to heal skin problems) (Saary et al. 2005) had been used in geophagia by pregnant women. Hunter (1984) reported the intake of 30 to 50 g of clays per day.

4.6 PROTECTION HYPOTHESIS

This hypothesis can also be termed the adaptive hypothesis:

> This hypothesis is based on the assumption that "geophagia substances have potential to adsorb microbial endotoxins and phytochemicals from the lumen of the gastrointestinal tract of humans."
>
> This adsorptive potential of clay, soil, kaolin, starch, and other pica materials is helpful in annulling harmful effects of ingested microbes and phytochemicals. Moreover, geophagia has detoxification properties. Humans are adapted to geophagia. This knowledge runs in families, communities, and tribes. It is transferred from one generation to another through its persistent practice among members of families. Consequently, the habit of geophagia assumes a cultural practice among the masses.
>
> Therefore, geophagia could be explained on the basis of a "protection-cum-adaptive hypothesis."

Another speculation is that pica materials can coat the epithelial surfaces of the gastrointestinal tract (GIT) and form a protective layer. This inhibits diffusion of endotoxins and phytochemicals from the lumen of the GIT into the inside of intestinal epithelial cells.

4.6.1 Descriptive Evidence in Favor of Protection Hypothesis

Clay eating among reptiles, birds, mammals, and non-chordates has been reported by Shachal et al. (1976) and Marlow and Tollestrup (1982). According to Mitchell et al. (1977) and Burchfield et al. (1977), clay eating among rats has been speculated to have evolved as a consequence of inflammation of the gut in response to phytochemicals.

Laufer (1930) mentioned literature citing the detoxification potential of geophagia against various chemicals like alkaloids, quinones, and tannins. The author reported clay eating among Native Americans of the American Southwest. The population habitually consumes clays, along with eating a wild variety of potatoes. Laufer

(1930) assumed it to be due to a detoxification property of clay through which it overcomes the bitter taste of potatoes and protects the inhabitants against the toxic effects of wild potatoes.

This assumption was supported by the work of Johns (1986), in which the author performed *in vitro* analysis of the adsorptive ability of clay. Johns (1986) observed that an alkaloid from wild potatoes was adsorbed by four different types of clay.

Another explanation for the adsorptive potential of clay and kaolin was provided by Dominy et al. (2004) in their *in vitro* research with a model of the human stomach and intestine. The models simulated the human stomach and intestine closely. The authors analyzed the ability of kaolin to adsorb quinine and tannin, and observed the reduction in bioavailability of materials due to reduced absorption of quinine and tannin.

> Dominy et al. (2004) concluded that adsorption of toxins by clay could be a relatively conceivable mechanism that accounts for the habit of geophagia.

According to other researchers (Johns and Duquette 1991), who analyzed the detoxification potential of different clays from Africa concomitant to the protection hypothesis of geophagia in humans, acorn has a bitter taste alkaloid called tannin acid. Johns and Duquette (1991) noted the maximum adsorptive ability of clays in Africa for tannic acid in ranges between 5.6 and 23.7 mg/g. They asserted African clays release minerals like calcium, copper, iron, zinc, and magnesium that have nutritional value for humans. Overall, the authors suggested that the habit of geophagia has a significance in the evolution of human dietary habits.

Still other researchers (Young et al. 2011) analyzed published papers related to hypotheses of geophagia in humans, mammals, birds, and reptiles. The authors concluded through their review that geophagia among humans was not associated with children and pregnant women. Young et al. (2011) also stated the absence of correlation between tropical areas and consumption of clay.

Moreover, Young et al. (2011) propounded that, linked to the intake of toxic substances and accompanied gut disturbance in primates, clay ingestion provided protection to primates from toxins and supplied nutrients. Importantly, the authors concluded that human clay intake was linked to protection from phytochemicals, microbes, and microbial endotoxins.

Another proponent of the protection hypothesis claimed that geophagy materials form a protective layer over the intestinal epithelium and confer resistance to invasion of pathogens and endotoxins (Hui et al. 2001).

Geophagia is practiced by women during pregnancy and children during periods of active growth. These physiological periods of human life need higher immunity against various biological and chemical stimuli. Ingestion of clay and starch during these periods confers protection against harmful stimuli and provides relief from microbial and/or chemical inflammation of the gut and associated nausea and vomiting.

Gardiner et al. (1993) studied the role of adsorbents in experimentally induced systemic endotoxemia in rat models. The release of endotoxins in the lumen of the gut disrupts the mucosal barrier and induces mucosal inflammation. Microbial toxins find a way into systemic circulation, causing endotoxaemia. The authors administered kaolin and terra fullonica orally. Gardiner et al. (1993) observed a reduction of system endotoxaemia; therefore, this study authenticates the use of clay and starch as materials of geophagia during pregnancy to reduce nausea and vomiting.

Krishnamani and Mahaney (2002) documented the presence of geophagia among primates either due to the antitoxic effect of geophagia, antacid action, anti-diarrheal effect, or the cumulative action of geophagia materials. Krishnamani and Mahaney (2002) concluded that primates habitually consume geophagia materials due to multiple factors.

In another study by Pebsworth et al. (2012), it was found that chacma baboons who were pregnant had greater proclivities for geophagia in comparison to other baboons who were not pregnant. Pebsworth et al. (2012) concluded that consumption of soils by pregnant chacma baboons might be helpful in relieving gastrointestinal discomfort.

Dominy et al. (2004) asserted that geophagia is an adaptive behavior in primates and other organisms. Clay and kaolin adsorb toxins from the intestine. Dominy et al. (2004) verified the hypothesis through *in vitro* analysis. Dominy et al. (2004) reported the reduction of bioavailability of quinine and tannins from the GIT.

Callahan (2003) reported the use of baked clay by select societies in the world, which could enhance immunity against pathogens. These baked clays are rich in aluminum salts. The formula of kaolin is $Al_2O_3\ 2SiO_2\ 2H_2O$ (Perry 2011).

According to Gupta (1998), aluminum salts are used as adjuvants with vaccines for humans. Adjuvants serve to improve the efficacy of vaccines and the immune response of the human body against pathogens. Aluminum adjuvants provide a surface for the adsorption of antigens. According to Gupta (1998), the adsorbed antigens on the surface of aluminum are rapidly taken up by antigen-presenting cells and promote rapid activation of the lymphocytes for immunity. Therefore, aluminum salts in vaccines and kaolin might promote the non-specific immune response of the body owing to their impact on dendritic cells, macrophages, and antigen-presenting cells.

Eating clays rich in aluminum salts in pregnancy by women could be a factor to enhance their immunity and provide innate immunity to the baby. According to Callahan (2003), clays could act as edible vaccines, and women consume clays in pregnancy. Clays might confer local immunity to a newborn baby through the suckling of milk that is enriched with immunoglobulin A due to the ingestion of clays (Callahan 2003).

According to Noguera-Obenza et al. (2002), the antibody IgA is secreted in mother's milk and provides mucosal immunity to the baby against endemic pathogens.

Clay eating in terms of the protection hypothesis can be construed as a means to induce local and systemic immunity in the body of pregnant women and confer mucosal immunity to newborn babies.

4.7 NEUROPSYCHIATRIC DISORDERS AND PICA

Pica might be associated with neuropsychiatric disorders like anxiety, depression, OCD, and developmental disability (Danford et al. 1982; Stiegler 2005; Stroman et al. 2011).

Cravings for non-food substances can be comparable to cravings for opium and alcohol, wherein both instances are associated with consumption alleviating psychological discomfort (Edwards et al. 1994; Young 2011).

Pica has been diagnosed as a feeding and eating disorder, according to the American Psychiatric Association's *Diagnostic and Statistical Manual of Mental Disorders, Fifth Edition* (Call et al. 2013; APA 2013).

Therefore, according to criteria suggested by the APA in the DSM-5 (2013), a pica habit can be represented by the following characteristics:

- Insistent consumption of non-food substances for a minimum duration of 1 month.

- Consumption of non-food substances should be unsuitable to the developmental status of the suffering individual.

- The eating behavior should be neither a cultural practice nor a socially supported behavior.

- If the eating behavior is associated with another mental disorder like autism, schizophrenia, or intellectual disability or occurs during a medical condition, including pregnancy, it requires immediate additional clinical examination.

Pica is generally associated with mental disorders that impair cognition, behavior, memory, and learning processes.

Luiselli (1996) observed the association of pica and geophagia with obsessive-compulsive disorder. Patients mentioned that pica was linked to their daily practices, rituals, and beliefs, and Luiselli (1996) reported a feeling of compulsion in the patients to practice pica.

4.7.1 Descriptive Evidence

Anorexia nervosa and bulimia nervosa are abnormal eating behaviors, and they are beset with psychopathological characteristics. Cnattingius et al. (1999) conducted a case-control and cohort study among girls to detect the association of anorexia nervosa with perinatal injury and gestational period. They found that girls with brain injury or cephalohematoma and those born alive before a gestational period of 28 to 32 weeks (very preterm birth) had higher odds of having an eating dysfunction like anorexia nervosa (Cnattingius et al. 1999).

Chipkevitch (1994) conducted a review of 21 cases through literature review. The author found that brain tumors coincided with clinical manifestations like anorexia nervosa, weight loss, and psychiatric symptoms in 19 cases (Chipkevitch 1994).

Carp (1950) observed that mentally deranged persons exhibited bizarre clinical symptoms as suicide attempts, injuring oneself, and ingestion of non-food substances of various sizes and shapes. Carp (1950) detected foreign bodies in the GITs of mentally deranged patients during surgical operations. Carp (1950) concluded that foreign bodies may accidentally find their way into the GIT. The author asserted that deliberate intake of foreign bodies is also seen in psychiatric patients.

Teinourian et al. (1964) indicated that ingestion of foreign bodies (non-food) is a frequent clinical manifestation among mentally deranged patients. It might be attributed to either the indiscriminate behavior of the patients or accidental intake of foreign bodies. Patients generally mask the signs and symptoms that arise from intake of foreign bodies. Additionally, Teinourian et al. (1964) described how this aberrant behavior among patients has a high rate of repetition. The author suggested that this behavior among psychiatric patients should be carefully attended (Teinourian et al. 1964).

Jacob et al. (1990) reported a case of a schizophrenic female patient who ingested foreign bodies that became lodged in the main bronchi, as revealed by radiographic examination of the chest of the patient after hospitalization. Jacob et al. (1990) reported the absence of foreign bodies in the GIT of the patient. The patient died due to cardiac arrest in the hospital.

Danford and Huber (1981) stated that eating dysfunctions like pica, hyperphagia, anorexia, and rumination are frequently observed in mentally retarded and mentally deranged patients.

Furthermore, the authors described that eating dysfunctions were associated with convulsions, level of intelligence, administration of drugs, and insomnia. Danford and Huber (1981) stated that eating dysfunctions like pica were associated with hyperphagia in patients and advised that eating dysfunctions must be carefully observed among patients, as these are associated with deficiency of macronutrients and micronutrients in the bodies of patients.

Cohen et al. (1976) described the habit of pica among children with abnormal development. Developmentally deranged children exhibited abnormal eating habits like geophagia, pica, and preference for other non-food substances. Cohen et al. (1976) observed the habit of lead ingestion among autistic children, and they detected high serum lead concentration in the bodies of autistic children when compared with normal children.

Herguner et al. (2008) asserted there was an association between geophagia and obsessive compulsive disorder.

Stein et al. (1996) studied the behavior of five patients with pica habits in clinics. The authors reported that two patients with pica presented the clinical manifestations of obsessive compulsive disorder. Patients responded to pharmacotherapy with serotonin reuptake inhibitors. Stein et al. (1996) documented that the habit of pica or geophagia in selected cases can be construed as compulsive behavior.

4.8 SUMMARY

- Geophagia is commonly practiced by women in pregnancy and by children, where both groups of patients have immune systems that are either suppressed in women or immature in children. The habit of clay eating could probably alleviate symptoms of gastritis in pregnant mothers and provide protection from microbial toxins to developing fetuses and children (Bogin et al. 2007; Ellis et al. 2009; Abrams and Miller 2011).

- Geophagia materials have a high affinity to cation exchange. They can strongly bind to pathogens, endotoxins, and phytotoxins. In this way, geophagy materials can reduce the bioavailability of toxins in the body and offer protection to humans (Johns 1986; Johns and Duquette 1991; Hooda et al. 2002).

- In amylophagia, raw rice contains a high amount of polysaccharides and proteins in the range of 80%–85% of carbohydrates and 6%–8% of proteins (USDA 2013). Consumption of raw rice may minimize iron absorption from the gut and help in preventing microbial infection in individuals. Raw rice may act like lactoferrins in the body of the host, which can limit bioavailability of iron for microbial proliferation (Fessler 2002). In this method, amylophagia could protect from pathogens.

- Geophagia materials like kaolin can adsorb bacterial toxins from the lumen of the alimentary canal in humans. Hence, kaolin ingestion could minimize mucosal inflammation and associated distress such as nausea and vomiting, which are common symptoms in the first trimester of pregnancy (Geissler et al. 1999).

- Micronutrients are elements that are required by organisms in trace amounts essential to sustain normal growth and development (UNICEF 2017; WHO and FAO 2004).

- The micronutrient deficiency hypothesis states, "Inadequacy of micronutrients is the prime etiological factor for the arousal of the physiological need that intensely motivates affected individuals to fulfill a micronutrient deficiency by adapting an aberrant behavior related to the eating of soil, clay, or any other earth-related non-food substances."

- The psychological stress hypothesis asserts that pica is a psychopathological disorder that arises in response to either external or internal psychological stress stimuli.

- The hunger hypothesis describes the habit of geophagia on the basis of the hunger drive in humans. Poverty, hunger, and starvation are the motivational forces to eat earth substances, like clay, soil, and kaolin, in the absence of adequate food sources in order to achieve a sense of satiety.

- According to Paul et al. (2015), culture is a social trait that underlies certain habits, practices, and discourses, which becomes the matrix for coherence and incoherence of social life over time. Geophagia, in certain societies of world, still persists as a cultural practice.

- The protection or adaptive hypothesis is based on the assumption that "geophagia substances have the potential to adsorb microbial endotoxins and phytochemicals from the lumen of the gastrointestinal tract of humans."

- Pica might be associated with neuropsychiatric disorders like anxiety, depression, OCD, and developmental disabilities (Danford et al. 1982; Stiegler 2005; Stroman et al. 2011).

- Cravings for non-food substances can be comparable to cravings for opium and alcohol, wherein both instances are associated with consumption alleviating psychological discomfort (Edwards et al. 1994, Young 2011).

- Schaller and Park (2011) hypothesized that in periods of risk of infection, the body defense mechanism in terms of behavior is modulated to adapt to the environment. In pregnancy, the immune system of the body is suppressed, leading to an altered behavior response in terms of nausea and vomiting. Geophagia in this phase of life might be a protective response against pathogens and toxins.

Conclusion

It is postulated that "geophagia among humans is a prehominid trait that has evolved as a behavioral adaptation to the physiological need for trace minerals coupled with protection from ingested microbial toxins that with the passage of time integrated with cultural practices."

REFERENCES

Abrahams PW, Parsons JA 1996. Geophagy in the tropics: A literature review. *The Geographical Journal* 162:63–72.

Abrams ET, Miller EM 2011. The roles of the immune system in women's reproduction: Evolutionary constraints and life history trade-offs. *Yearb Phys Anthropol* 54:134–154.

American Psychiatric Association 2013. Feeding and eating disorders. In: *Diagnostic and Statistical Manual of Mental Disorders*. 5th ed. pp. 329–331.

American Psychological Association 2013. *Diagnostic Statistical Manual of Mental Disorders: DSM-V*. Washington D. C.: American Psychological Association.

Arcasoy A, Cavdar A, Babacan E 1978. Ferrokinetic studies in patients with geophagia, growth retardation, hypogonadism, hepatosplenomegaly, iron deficiency anemia, and zinc deficiency. *Acta Haematol* 60:76–84.

Artur L, Hilhorst D 2014. Floods, resettlement and land access and use in the lower Zambezi, Mozambique. *Land Use Policy* 36:361–368.

Barton JC, Barton C, Bertoli LF 2016. Pica for uncooked basmati rice in two women with iron deficiency and a review of ryzophagia. *Case Rep Med* 2016:5.

Bateson EM, Lebroy T 1978. Clay eating by aboriginals of the Northern Territory. *Med J Aust* 1(Suppl 1):1–3.

BBC News 2016. The people who can't stop eating dirt. BBC News. 16 June 2016.

Beard JL, Chen Q, Connor J, Jones BC 1994. Altered monamine metabolism in caudate-putamen of iron-deficient rats. *Pharmacol Biochem Behav* 48:621–624.

Benno S, Ara A, eds. 2009. Dirt poor haitians eat mud cookies to survive. Huffington Post. Retrieved 9 August 2015.

Berridge KC, Kringelbach ML 2015. Pleasure systems in the brain. *Neuron* 86(3):646–664.

Bhan MK, Sommerfelt H, Strand T 2001. Micronutrient deficiency in children. *Br J Nutr* 85(Suppl 2):S199–S203.

Bhatia MS, Gupta R 2009. Pica responding to SSRI and OPD spectrum disorder? *World J Biol Psychiatry* 10(4):936–938.

Bianco LE, Wiesinger J, Earley CJ, Jones BC, Beard JL 2008. Iron deficiency alters dopamine uptake and response to L-DOPA injection in Sprague-Dawley rats. *J Neurochem* 106:205–215.

Bithoney WG, Snyder J, Michalek J, Newberger EH 1985. Childhood ingestions as symptoms of family distress. *Am J Dis Child* 13(9): 456–459.

Black RE 2001. Micronutrients in pregnancy. *Br J Nutr* 85:S193–S197.

Blinder B, Goodman S, Henderson P 1988. Pica: A critical review of diagnosis and treatment. In: Blinder B, Chaitin B, Goldstein R, editors. *The Eating Disorders: Medical and Psychological Bases of Diagnosis and Treatment*. PMA Publishing Corp: New York, pp. 331–344.

Bogin B, Silva MIV, Rios L 2007. Life history trade-offs in human growth: Adaptation or pathology? *Am J Hum Biol* 19:631–642.

Bourne JK 2008. Dirt poor. Haiti has lost its soil-and the means to feed itself. *Natl Geo Mag* 214(3): 108–111.

Brand C, Jager LD, Ekosse GI 2009a. Health and social impacts of geophagy in Panama. *J Med Technol* 23:11–13.

Burchfield SR, Elich MS, Woods SC 1977. Geophagia in response to stress and arthritis. *Physiol & Behav* 19:265–267.

Butterley J, Sheperd J 2010. *Hunger: The Biology and Politics of Starvation*. Dartmouth College Press, Hanover, NH.

Calabresi P, Picconi B, Tozzi A, Ghiglieri V, Di Filippo M 2014. Direct and indirect pathways of basal ganglia: A critical reappraisal. *Nat Neurosci* 17:1022–1030.

Call C, Walsh BT, Attia E 2013. From DSM-IV to DSM-5: Changes to eating disorder diagnoses. *Curr Opin Psychiatry* 26:532–536.

Callahan GN 2003. Eating dirt. *Emerg Infect Dis* 9(8):1016–1021.

Cambridge English dictionary 2017. Meaning of Culture. Available at: http://dictionary.cambridge.org/dictionary/english/culture?a=british

Campbell DI, Murch SH, Elia M, Sullivan PB, Sanyang MS, Jobarteh B, Lunn PG 2003a. Canadian UNICEF Committee (2006) Global Child Survival and Health. p. 67.

Campbell DI, Murch SH, Elia M, Sullivan PB, Sanyang MS, Jobarteh B, Lunn PG 2003b. Chronic T cell-mediated enteropathy in rural west African children: Relationship with nutritional status and small bowel function. *Pediatr Res* 54:306–311.

Carp L 1950. Foreign bodies in the gastrointestinal tracts of psychotic patients. *Arch Surg* 60:1055–1075.

Carretero M 2002. Clay minerals and their beneficial effects upon human health. *A review Appl Clay Sci* 21:155–163

Castro J, Boyd-Orr J 1952. *The Geography of Hunger*. Little, Brown and Company, Boston.

Cavdar AO, Arcasoy A, Cin S, Babacon E, Gözdasoğlu S 1983. Geophagia in Turkey: Iron and zinc deficiency, iron and zinc absorption studies and response to treatment with zinc in geophagia cases. *Prog Clin Biol Res* 129:71–97.

Chipkevitch E 1994. Brain tumors and anorexia nervosa syndrome. *Brain Dev* 6:175–179.

Chokhi Dhani 2014. Haldighati. Available at: https://www.chokhidhani.com/village/haldighati

Christian P 2010. Micronutrients, birth weight, and survival. *Annu Rev Nutr* 30:83–104.

Cnattingius S, Hultman CM, Dahl M, Sparen P 1999. Very preterm birth, birth trauma, and the risk of anorexia nervosa among girls. *Arch Gen Psychiatry* 56:634–638.

Cohen DF, Johnson WT, Caparulo BK 1976. Pica and elevated blood lead level in autistic and atypical children. *Am J Dis Child* 130:47–48.

Cooskey NR 1995. Pica and olfactory craving of pregnancy: How deep are the secrets? *Birth* 22:129–136.

Corbett J 1988. Famine and household coping strategies. *World Dev* 16:1099–1112.

Crosby WH 1976. Pica: A compulsion caused by iron deficiency. *Br J Hematol* 34:341–342.

Cross NA, Hillman LS, Allen SH, Krause GF, Vieira NE 1995. Calcium homeostasis and bone metabolism during pregnancy, lactation, and post weaning: A longitudinal study. *Am J Clin Nutr* 61(3):514–523.

Danford DE, Huber AM 1981. Eating dysfunctions in an institutionalized mentally retarded population. *Appetite* 2:281–292.

Danford DE, Smith S, Huber A 1982. Pica and mineral status in mentally retarded. *Am J Clin Nutr* 35:958–967.

Darnton-Hill L, Mkparu UC 2015. Micronutrients in pregnancy in low- and middle-income countries. *Nutrients* 7(3):1744–1768.

Dhonukshe-Rutten RA, Bouwman J, Brown KA, Cavelaars AE, Collings R, Grammatikaki E, de Groot LC, Gurinovic M, Harvey LJ, Hermoso M 2013. EURRECA—Evidence-based methodology for deriving micronutrient recommendations. *Crit Rev Food Sci Nutr* 53:999–1040.

Dominy NJ, Davoust E, Minekus M 2004. Adaptive function of soil consumption: An *in vitro* study modeling the human stomach and small intestine. *J Exp Biol* 207(2):319–324.

Edwards CH, Johnson AA, Knight EM 1994. Pica in an urban environment. *J Nutr* 124(6 Suppl):954S–962S.

Ellis B, Figueredo AJ, Brumbach BH, Schlomer GL 2009. Fundamental dimensions of environmental risk: The impact of harsh versus unpredictable environments on the evolution of development of life history strategies. *Hum Nat* 20:204–268.

Ferré S, Lluís C, Justinova Z, Quiroz C, Orru M, Navarro G, Canela EI, Franco R, Goldberg SR 2010. Adenosine-cannabinoid receptor interactions. Implications for striatal function. *Br J Pharmacol* 160(3):443–453.

Fessler DT 2002. Reproductive immunosuppression and diet. *Curr Anthropol* 43:19–61.

Food and Agriculture Organization of the United Nations 2005. What Is Meant by Term "Quality of Food?" Available at: http://foodqualityschemes.jrc.es/en/documents/Finalreport_000.pdf

Food and Agricultural Organization of United Nations 2018. (Retrieved 2019) Food Security and Nutrition around the World. Available at: http://www.fao.org/state-of-food-security-nutrition/en/

Frate DA 1984. Last of the earth eaters. *Sciences* 24:34–38.

Gardiner KR, Anderson NH, McCaigue MD, Erwin PJ, Halliday MI 1993. Adsorbents as antiendotoxin agents in experimental colitis. *Gut* 34:51–55.

Geissler PW, Prince RJ, Levene M, Poda C, Beckerleg SE, Muteni W, Shulman CE 1999. Perceptions of soil-eating and anaemia among pregnant women on the Kenyan coast. *Soc Sci Med*, 48(8):1069–1079.

Geissler PW 2000. The significance of earth-eating: Social and cultural aspects of geophagy among Luo children. *Africa* 70(4):653–682.

Gelfand M 1945. Geophagy and its relation to hookworm disease. *East Afr Med J* 22:98–103.

Gernand AD, Schulze KJ, Stewart CP, West KP Jr, Christian P 2016. Micronutrient deficiencies in pregnancy worldwide: Health effects and prevention. *Nat Rev Endocrinol* 12(5):274–289.

Goldstein M 1998. Adult pica: A clinical nexus of physiology and psychodynamics. *Psychosomatics* 39(5):465–469.

Gregory JR 1995. *National Diet and Nutrition Survey in Children Ages 1.5–4.5 Years.* HMSO, London.

Grigsby RK, Thyer BA, Waller RJ, Johnston GA Jr 1999. Chalk eating in middle Georgia: A culture-bound syndrome of pica? *South Med J* 92(2):190–192.

Gupta A 2015. To analyze effect of pallor (anemia) on nutritional status of children under age of five years. *Gold Res Thoughts J* 4(7):1–9.

Gupta RK 1998. Aluminum compounds as vaccine adjuvants. *Adv Drug Rev* 32(3):155–172.

Hadley C, Crooks DL 2012. Coping and the biosocial consequences of food insecurity in the 21st century. *Yearb Phys Anthropol* 149(S55):72–94.

Hawass NED, Alnozha MM, Kolawole T 1987. Adult geophagia— Report of three cases with review of the literature. *Trop Geogr Med* 39:191–195.

Herguner S, Ozyildirim I, Tanidir C 2008. Is pica an eating disorder or an obsessive-compulsive spectrum disorder? *Prog Neuropsychopharmacol Biol Psychiatry* 32(12):2010–2011.

Hooda PS, Henry CJK, Seyoum TA, Armstrong LDM, Fowler MB 2002. Bioavailability of iron in geophagic earths and clay minerals, and their effect on dietary iron absorption using an *in vitro* digestion/ Caco-2 cell model. *Environ Geochem Health* 24:305–319.

Horner RD, Lackey CJ, Kolasa K, Warren K 1991. Pica practices of pregnant women. *J Am Diet Assoc* 91:34–39.

Hui YH, Smith RA, Spoerke DG 2001. *Foodborne Disease Handbook.* Vol. 1: Diseases Caused by Bacteria. Marcel Dekker, Inc., New York.

Hunter BT 2004. *Soil and Your Health: Healthy Soil Is Vital to Your Health.* Hirsch T (editor), Basic Health Publication Inc., North Bergen.

Hunter JM 1973. Geophagy in Africa and in the United States: A culture nutrition hypothesis. *Geogr Rev* 63:170–195.

Hunter JM 1984. Insect clay geophagy in Sierra Leone. *J Cult Geogr* 4:2–3.

International Food Policy Research Institute 2014. *Global Nutrition Report 2014.* International Food Policy Research Institute, Washington, DC.

Jacob B, Huckenbeck W, Barz J, Bonte W 1990. Death, after swallowing and aspiration of a high number of foreign bodies, in a schizophrenic woman. *Am J Forensic Med Pathol* 11(4):331–335.

James JA 1989. Preventing iron deficiency anaemia in pre-school children by implementing an educational and screening programme in an inner-city practice. *BMJ* 299:838–840.

Ji Hyun K, Antonio PS 2012. Dopaminergic neurotransmission in the human brain: New lessons from perturbation and imaging. *Neuroscientist* 18(2): 149–168.

Johns T 1986. Detoxification function of geophagy and domestication of the potato. *J Chem Ecol* 12(3):635–646.

Johns T 1990. *With Bitter Herbs They Shall Eat It: Chemical Ecology and the Origins of Human Diet and Medicine.* University of Arizona Press, Tucson, AZ.

Johns T, Duquette M 1991. Detoxification and mineral supplementation as functions of geophagy. *Am J Clin Nutr* 53:448–456.

Johnson BE 1990. Pica. In: Walker HK, Hall WD, Hurst JW, editors. *Clinical Methods: The History, Physical, and Laboratory Examinations.* 3rd ed. Butterworths; Boston.

Katz DL 2008. *Diet, Pregnancy and Lactation. Nutrition in Clinical Practice.* Lippincott Williams & Wilkins, Philadelphia, pp. 299–309.

Kravitz AV, Freeze BS, Parker PR, Kay K, Thwin MT, Deisseroth K, Kreitzer AC 2010. Regulation of Parkinsonian motor behaviours by optogenetic control of basal ganglia circuitry. *Nature* 466:622–626.

Krishnamani R, Mahaney WC 2002. Geophagy among primates: Adaptive significance and ecological consequences. *Anim Behav* 59:899–915.

Lacey EP 1990. Pica: Consideration of a historical and current problem with racial/ethnic/cultural overtones. *Explor Ethn Stud* 12(1):1–8.

Ladipo OA 2000. Nutrition in pregnancy: Mineral and vitamin supplements. *Am J Clin Nutr* 72(1): 280S–290S.

Laufer B 1930. *Geophagy.* Publication 280, Anthropology Series, 18(2): Chicago: Field Museum of Natural History.

Luiselli JK 1996. Pica as an obsessive-compulsive disorder. *J Behav Ther Exp Psychiat* 27(2):195–196.

Luoba AI, Geissler PW, Estambale B, Ouma JH, Magnussen P, Alusala D, Ayah R, Mwaniki D, Friis H 2004. Geophagy among pregnant and lactating women in Bondo District, western Kenya. *Trans R Soc Trop Med Hyg* 98:734–741.

Malenka RC, Nestler EJ, Hyman SE 2009. Widely Projecting Systems: Monoamines, Acetylcholine, and Orexin. In: Sydor A, Brown RY (eds.). *Molecular Neuropharmacology: A Foundation for Clinical Neuroscience* (2nd ed.). New York: McGraw-Hill Medical. pp. 147–148, 154–157.

Marlow RW, Tollestrup K 1982. Mining and exploitation of natural mineral deposits by the desert tortoise, *Gopherus agassizii*. *Anim Behav* 30:475–478.

Maslow AH 1943. A theory of human motivation. *Psychological Review* 50(4):370–396.

Mitchell D, Laycock JD, Stephens WF 1977. Motion sickness-induced pica in the rat. *Am J Clin Nutr* 30:147–150.

Montague PR, Dayan P, Sejnowski TJ 1996. A framework for mesencephalic dopamine systems based on predictive Hebbian learning. *J Neurosci* 16:1936–1947.

Moore SF, Puritt P 1977. *The Chagga and Meeru of Tanzania. Ethnographic survey of Africa, East Central Africa*. International African Institute.

Morton L 1953. *The fall of the Philippines*. United States Army Hospital, History, pp. 171–202.

Moser C 1996. *Confronting crisis: A comparative study of household responses to poverty and vulnerability in four poor urban communities*. Washington, DC: World Bank.

Mridula D, Mishra CP, Chakraverty A 2003. Dietary intake of expectant mother. *Indian J Nutr Diet* 40(1):24–30.

National Research Council (NRC) 1986. *Nutrient Adequacy: Assessment Using Food Consumption Surveys*. Washington, DC: The National Academies Press. Available at: https://www.ncbi.nlm.nih.gov/books/NBK217533/

Ngozi PO 2008. Pica practices of pregnant women in Nairobi, Kenya. *East Afr Med J* 85(2):72–79.

Njiru H, Elchalal U, Paltiel O 2011. Geophagy during pregnancy in Africa: A literature review. *Obstet Gynecol Surv* 66:452–459.

Noguera-Obenza M, Ochoa TJ, Gomez HF, Guerrero ML, Herrera-Insua I, Morrow AL 2002. Human milk secretory antibodies against attaching and effacing *Eschericia coli* antigens. *Emerg Infect Dis* 9:545–555.

Paul J, Liam M, Andy S, Steger MB 2015. *Urban Sustainability in Theory and Practice: Circles of Sustainability*. Routledge, London, p. 53.

Pebsworth PA, Bardi M, Huffman MA 2012. Geophagy in chacma baboons: Patterns of soil consumption by age class, sex, and reproductive state. *Am J Primatol* 74(1):48–57.

Perry DL 2011. *Handbook of Inorganic Compounds*. Taylor & Francis.

Ray N 2002. Lonely Planet Cambodia. Lonely Planet Publication, p. 308. Available at: https://en.wikipedia.org/wiki/Fried_spider

Robert PH 2013. Dairy intake, dietary adequacy, and lactose intolerance. *Adv Nutr* 4(2):151–156.

Rose EA, Porcerelli JH, Neale AV 2000. Pica: Common but commonly missed. *J Am Board Fam Pract* 13:353–8

Rwegerera GM, Joel DR, Bakilana C, Maruza MP 2015. The triad of iron deficiency anemia, hepatosplenomegaly and growth retardation with normal serum zinc levels in a 14-year-old boy. *Niger J Clin Pract* 18(5):690–692.

Saary J, Qureshi R, Palda V, Dekoven J, Pratt M, Skotnicki-Grant S, Holness L 2005. A systematic review of contact dermatitis treatment and prevention. *J Am Acad Dermatol* 53(5):845.

Schaller M, Park J 2011. The behavioral immune system (and why it matters). *Curr Dir Psychol Sci* 20:99–103.

Schultz W 1998. Predictive reward signal of dopamine neurons. *J Neurophysiol* 80:1–27.

Schultz W 2015. Neuronal reward and decision signals: From theories to data. *Physiol Rev* 95(3):853–951.

Selye H 1956. *The Stress of Life*. McGraw-Hill, New York.

Shachal EA, Chapman Y, Steinberger Y 1976. Feeding, energy flow and soil turnover in the desert isopod, *Hemilepistus reaumuri*. *Oecologia* 24:57–69.

Shipton P 1990. African famines and food security: Anthropological perspectives. *Annu Rev Anthropol* 19:353–394.

Singhi S, Ravishanker R, Singhi P, Nath R 2003. Low plasma zinc and iron in pica. *Indian J Pediatr* 70:139–143.

Singhi S, Singhi P, Adwani GB 1981. Role of psychosocial stress in the cause of pica. *Clin Pediatr* 20:783–785.

Stein DJ, Bouwer C, van Heerden B 1996. Pica and the obsessive-compulsive spectrum disorders. *S Afr Med J* 86(12l):1586–1588.

Stiegler L 2005. Understanding pica behavior: A review for clinical and educational professionals. *Focus Autism Other Dev Disabil* 20:27–38.

Stroman D, Young C, Rubano AR, Pinkhasov A 2011. *Adult-onset pica leading to acute intestinal obstruction*. *Psychosomatics* 52(4):393–394. doi: 10.1016/j.psym.2011.01.031.

Sugita K 2001. Pica: Pathogenesis and therapeutic approach. *Nippon Rinsho* 59(3):561–565.

Taylor SB, Lewis CR, Olive MF 2013. The neurocircuitry of illicit psychostimulant addiction: Acute and chronic effects in humans. *Subst Abuse Rehabil* 4:29–43.

Teinourian B, Cigtay AS, Smyth NP 1964. Management of ingested foreign bodies in the psychotic patient. *Arch Surg* 88:915–920.

Thompson B, Amoroso L (editors) 2014. *Improving Diets and Nutrition: Food-Based Approaches.* FAO and CAB International, Rome and Wallingford.

Tritsch NX, Sabatini BL 2012. Dopaminergic modulation of synaptic transmission in cortex and striatum. *Neuron* 76:33–50.

Unger EL, Bianco LE, Jones BC, Allen RP, Earley CJ 2014. Low brain iron effects and reversibility on striatal dopamine dynamics. *Exp Neurol* 261:462–468.

UNICEF 2017. Micronutrients and Hidden Hunger. Available at: https://www.unicef.org/republicadominicana/english/survival_development_12473.htm

United States Department of Agriculture, National Institute of Food and Agriculture (Retrieved 2019) Food Quality. Available at: https://nifa.usda.gov/topic/food-quality

United States Department of Agriculture 2013. National Agricultural Library. Available at: http://ndb.nal.usda.gov. Accessed 2017.

United States Department of Agriculture 2017. *Vitamins and Minerals.* National Agricultural Library.

Van Huis A 1996. The traditional use of arthropods in Sub Saharan Africa. *Proc Exp Appl Entomol* 7:3–20.

van Vliet S, Burd NA, van Loon LJ 2015. The skeletal muscle anabolic response to plant- versus animal-based protein consumption. *J Nutr* 145(9):1981–1991.

Vermeer DE 1966. Geophagy among the TIV of Nigeria. *Ann Assoc Am Geogr* 56:197–204.

Wasantwisut E 1997. Nutrition and development: Other micronutrient' effect on growth and cognition. Southeast Asian. *J Trop Med Public Health* 28 Suppl., 2:78–82.

Wiley AS, Solomon HK 1998. Geophagy in pregnancy: A test of a hypothesis. *Curr Anthropol* 39:532–545.

World Health Organization (WHO), Food and Agricultural Organization (FAO) of the United Nations 2004. Vitamin and mineral requirements in human nutrition. Available at: https://www.who.int/nutrition/publications/micronutrients/9241546123/en/

World Health Organization 2017a. Nutrition: Micronutrients. Available at: http://www.who.int/nutrition/topics/micronutrients/en/

World Health Organization 2017. Nutrition: What Is Hidden Hunger? Available at: http://www.who.int/nutrition/topics/WHO_FAO_ICN2_videos_hiddenhunger/en/

Yager LM, Garcia AF, Wunsch AM, Ferguson SM 2015. The ins and outs of the striatum: Role in drug addiction. *Neuroscience* 301:529–541.

Young SL 2010. Pica in pregnancy: New ideas about an old condition. *Annu Rev Nutr* 30:403–422.

Youdim MB, Ashkenazi R, Ben-Shachar D, Yehuda S 1984. Modulation of dopamine receptor in the striatum by iron: Behavioral and biochemical correlates. *Adv Neurol* 40:159–170.

Youdim MB, Ben-Shachar D, Ashkenazi R, Yehuda S 1983. Brain iron and dopamine receptor function. *Adv Biochem Psychopharmacol* 37:309–321.

Young SL 2011. *Craving Earth: Understanding Pica: The Urge to Eat Clay, Starch, Ice, and Chalk.* Columbia University Press, New York.

Young SL, Sherman PW, Lucks JB, Pelto GH 2011. Why on earth?: Evaluating hypotheses about the physiological functions of human geophagy. *Q Rev Biol* 86(2):97–120.

Yves G, Dechassa L 2000. Wild Food Plants in Southern Ethiopia: Reflections on the Role of Famine-Foods at a Time of Drought. UN-OCHA Report. Available at: https://en.wikipedia.org/wiki/Famine_food

Zalilah MS, Ang M 2001. Assessment of food insecurity among low income households in Kuala Lumpur using the Radimer/Cornell food insecurity instrument—A validation study. *Malays J Nutr* 7:15–32.

Zalilah MS, Tham BL 2002. Food security and child nutritional status among Orang Asli (Temuan) households in Hulu Langat, Selangor. *Med J Malaysia* 57:36–50.

Zedlitz K. 2010. Pica—A historical "eating disorder". *Wurzbg Medizinhist Mitt* 29:402–433.

CHAPTER **5**

Ill Effects of Geophagia on Nutritional Status of Preschool Children

MALNUTRITION NEGATIVELY AFFECTS GROWTH during intrauterine life as well as invariably disturbing the growth of the baby in postnatal life. It is manifested as a deficiency in the weight and/or height of a child according to his or her age. The deficiency of minerals in the body of children in the formative years of life is intensely implicated in malnutrition. Micronutrient inadequacy is closely linked to higher susceptibility to acquire infections, delayed recovery from infections, and frequent relapse of infections in children, thereby resulting in a high child mortality rate. According to Black et al. (2013) and Brennhofer et al. (2017), about 25% of the child mortality in the world is attributed to malnutrition; in other words, it is asserted by the authors that around 3.1 million children die annually due to poor nutrition.

According to studies conducted by Geissler et al. (1998) and Ngure et al. (2013) in Zimbabwe and Kenya, geophagia was associated with a greater tendency toward helminthic infestation and environmental enteropathy in children who practiced it. A study by George et al. (2015) described the ill effects of geophagia that manifested in the form of inflammation of intestinal mucosa, malabsorption syndrome, and stunting among children. Further, the authors concluded there was insufficient information concerning the quantity, frequency, and type of soil ingested by the affected population of children.

Perin et al. (2016), in a study in rural Bangladesh, described a relationship between geophagia and enteric infection in children who were afflicted with soil eating. This could lead to malnutrition. Perin et al. (2016) conducted a prospective cohort study composed of 216 children below the age of 5 years. The authors observed growth deficits in children who were involved in geophagia. They described deficiencies in the weight and height of affected children in comparison to those who were not addicted to the habit of soil eating. Perin et al. (2016) reported a prevalence of 21% of stunting in children.

In the formative years, children pass through an oral stage and try to explore objects by putting them in the mouth, which is considered normal development. However, the soil that is ingested by a child in the act of exploration becomes injurious owing to its contaminants like worms, heavy metals, and other particulate matter that could damage the mucosa of the alimentary canal (Shivoga and Moturi 2009).

Gupta (2015a, b) conducted a study in Fazilka city in the Punjab state in India. The study was composed of children from 2 years to under 5 years of age who resided in Fazilka. Children who were sick and uncooperative in physical examination were excluded from the study by the author. A sample size of 382 was estimated, and a non-response rate of 10% was computed, which, when added, resulted in a sample size of 440 children. The author undertook a descriptive cohort study. The structure of the sample showed children (240/440) selected from schools, those (127/440) selected from anganwadi, and the remaining children (73/440) selected from slum areas. The author analyzed the data that originated from the study by physical examination, anthropometric examination, and personal interviews with caretakers, teachers, and parents of children. The author described a prevalence of 9.4% (41/440) of geophagia in the children, and posited that geophagia exhibited fluctuation according to age groups as a 20.2% prevalence of geophagia in the 2- to 3-year age group, while the prevalence was 1.6% in children >3 to <5 years.

The author calculated the odds ratio (OR) to analyze the presence of wasting among children who were addicted to geophagia in comparison to children who were healthy (geophagia absent). The author found a high odds ratio (22.89) at significance level $p < 0.0001$ between the habit of geophagy and wasting in children. The author concluded that the habit of geophagia among children at the tender age of under 5 years increases manyfold the probability of malnutrition (wasting) in children.

Gupta (2017) conducted a descriptive study among children below the age of 5 years in the city of Fazilka. The study was composed of 440 children in the age group between 2 years and under 5 years. The author described that 41 children were affected with the habit of geophagia, with a prevalence of 9.4%. The remaining children ($n = 399$) were healthy and without the habit of geophagia. Further, the author posited that about 51% ($n = 21$) of the geophagia-afflicted children ($n = 41$) suffered from stunting. Again, the author described that some of the children ($n = 105$) out of the total number of children ($n = 399$) who were without the habit of geophagia also suffered from stunting. Therefore, non-geophagia children showed a prevalence of 26% of stunting. The author conducted a bivariate, inferential analysis of the data and described 2.9 times higher odds of stunting in children who practiced geophagia in comparison to children who did not have the habit of geophagia.

Gupta (2015a,b), in another study, described the ill effects of geophagia on the affected preschool children. The author observed that pallor was significantly detected upon physical examination of the children who had the habit of geophagia. In a statistical analysis, the author found that the possibility of the presence of pallor was 85 times higher [geophagy and pallor, OR = 0.527/0.0062 = (85.64) 95%, CI (20.22–362.6)] in children who practiced geophagia in comparison to those who were healthy and without the habit of geophagia. This was explored by computing the odds ratio. This compared the odds of pallor in the presence of geophagy, the predictor variable, with those of the absence of geophagy. The odds ratio between poor growth during infancy and early childhood remains an important risk factor for childhood morbidity and mortality and a major public health challenge in low- and middle-income countries. Childhood stunting is a risk factor for diminished survival, short adult height, impaired intellectual development, reduced economic productivity, and offspring with low birth weight.

Globally, approximately 178 million children less than 5 years of age are stunted, with an estimated 35% of child deaths attributed to suboptimal nutrition.

Environmental enteropathy is a disorder of the intestinal mucosa and is characterized by its chronic inflammation. This disorder is prevalent in the child population residing in poor settings. According to Solomons (2003; Black et al. 2018), it is a leading cause of stunting among children in developing countries. It is manifested as low localized immunity of the gut and chronic inflammation. According to Humphrey (2009), environmental enteropathy is the second most important cause of growth deficits among children. The habit of geophagia predisposes children to environmental enteropathy and malnutrition. Solomons (2003) postulated uncertainty of the etiology of environmental enteropathy; nonetheless, it is associated with poor sanitation, unsafe drinking water, and unhygienic practices in daily life. These conditions predispose the fecal-oral route of infection (Wagner and Lanoix 1958). The authors described food, fluids, house flies, and fingers in the spread of infection in the fecal-oral route.

Conclusion

- Authors, historians, clinicians, and anthropologists agree universally that geophagia is a global phenomenon.
- The habit of geophagia exhibits adaptive potential among humans.
- Geophagia is an aberrant eating behavior that has myriad causal factors in its pathogenesis that in turn interplay. The factors could be classified into two main categories, biological and cultural.
- Geophagia has a strong cultural underpinning that is evident from the fact that it is deeply instilled in societies in the form of rituals and beliefs. Therefore, geophagia has been labeled a "cultural institution" by Hunter, especially in the African subcontinent.
- Extensive cross-cultural data are essential to understand the exact role of geophagia in human civilization. Data should be collected from the part of the world where it is strongly prevalent. The daily life of inhabitants should be monitored. Geophagia samples should be investigated. The age and gender predilection of geophagia should be explored. The roles of natural calamity, food policy of a nation, food security, and population density should be studied to pinpoint the exact cause of geophagia among humans.

REFERENCES

Black RE, Allen LH, Bhutta ZA, Caulfield LE, Onis M, Ezzati M, Mathers C, Rivera J 2008. Maternal and child undernutrition: Global and regional exposures and health consequences. *Lancet* 371:243–260.

Black RE, Victora CG, Walker SP, Bhutta ZA, Christian P, de Onis M 2013. Maternal and child undernutrition and overweight in low-income and middle-income countries. *Lancet* 382:427–451.

Brennhofer S, Reifsnider E, Bruening M 2017. Malnutrition coupled with diarrheal and respiratory infections among children in Asia: A systematic review. *Public Health Nurs* 34(4):401–409.

Geissler PW, Mwaniki D, Thiong F, Friis H 1998. Geophagy as a risk factor for geohelminth infections: A longitudinal study of Kenyan primary schoolchildren. *Trans R Soc Trop Med Hyg* 92:7–11.

George CM, Oldja L, Biswas S, Perin J, Lee GO, Kosek M 2015. Geophagy is associated with environmental enteropathy and stunting in children in rural Bangladesh. *Am J Trop Med Hyg* 92:1117–1124.

Gupta A 2015a. Detrimental consequences of the habit of geophagy in children under the age of five years. *Rev Res J* 4(4):1–9.

Gupta A 2015b. Effect of geophagia on the nutritional status of children under five years of age. *Indian Streams Res J* 4(12).

Gupta A 2017. Assessing stunting and predisposing factors among children. *Asian J Pharm Clin Res* 10(10):1–8.

Humphrey JH 2009. Child undernutrition, tropical enteropathy, toilets, and hand washing. *Lancet* 374:1032–1035.

Ngure FM, Humphrey JH, Mbuya MN, Majo F, Mutasa K, Govha M 2013. Formative research on hygiene behaviors and geophagy among infants and young children and implications of exposure to fecal bacteria. *Am J Trop Med Hyg* 89:709–716.

Perin J, Thomas A, Oldja L, Ahmed S, Parvin T, Islam Bhuyian S 2016. Geophagy is associated with growth faltering in children in rural Bangladesh. *J Pediatr* 178:34–39.

Shivoga WA, Moturi WN 2009. Geophagia as a risk factor for diarrhoea. *J Infect Dev Ctries* 3:94–98.

Solomons NW 2003. Environmental contamination and chronic inflammation influence human growth potential. *J Nutr* 13:1237.

Wagner EG, Lanoix J 1958. *Excreta Disposal for Rural Areas and Small Countries*. WHO Monograph Series No. 39. World Health Organization, Geneva.

Index